KNOW YOUR

MEDICINES

This book is to be
or before the date st

Pat Blair

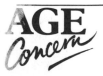

BOOKS

©1985, 1991, 1997 Pat Blair
1991 Revised edition
1997 Revised edition

Published by Age Concern England
1268 London Road
London SW16 4ER

Editor Gillian Clarke
Design and typesetting GreenGate Publishing Services
Production Vinnette Marshall
Printed and bound in Great Britain by Bell & Bain Ltd, Glasgow

A catalogue record for this book is available from the British Library.

ISBN 0–86242–226–4

Bulk orders
Age Concern England is pleased to offer customised editions of all its titles to UK companies, institutions or other organisations wishing to make a bulk purchase. For further information, please contact the Publishing Department at the address on this page. Tel: 0181-679 8000. Fax: 0181-679 6069. E-mail: addisom@ace.org.uk

Contents

Your Defence Systems

What medicines do: *including allergy to drugs used to treat infections, groups of drugs used to treat infections, vaccines*

SECTION 3: FURTHER INFORMATION

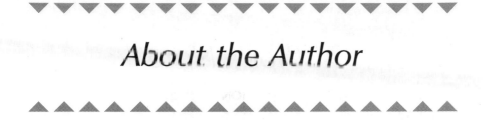

About the Author

Pat Blair, born and educated in Edinburgh, has specialised in medical journalism for twenty years. Now a freelance journalist and author, she is a contributor both to the national press and to publications aimed at those working in health and social care. A former chairman of the Medical Journalists' Association, she lives with her husband and family in London.

Author's Note

This is a guide to medicines for older people and those who help to care for them. It also explains how the body works and how it is affected by drugs. The medicines explained are those that you may buy or are prescribed by a doctor for you to take at home. Medicines generally administered in hospitals and clinics, or those such as injections that a doctor or nurse may give you at home, are not included. Where appropriate, medicines are listed by their recommended International Nonproprietary Name (rINN) but the British Approved Name (BAN) has also been retained (in brackets).

Section 1 of the book gives general information about using medicines, and is a guide to questions to ask your doctor or pharmacist. More details about this section are in the Contents on pages iii and iv.

Section 2 is divided into chapters broadly based on the actions of medicines on your body systems. It contains information on the common ailments affecting older people and many of the drugs used to treat them. There is no separate chapter dealing with the reproductive system, which is covered in the chapters on the glandular and urinary systems.

Section 3 includes an index where you can look up the names of the medicines that you have bought or been prescribed, to check what they are for and what they do. Even if the medicine you take is not included, the book should still be a useful general guide. Because it is not a guide to self-diagnosis and treatment, symptoms and ailments are not indexed separately.

Acknowledgements

In producing this third edition, I am indebted – once more – to colleagues, friends and acquaintances in the medical and allied professions who provided useful comment and suggested amendments, and without whose advice and guidance this book would never have been written. I am continually grateful to those older friends and relatives who have suffered my questions and who have been so helpful with their answers. Finally, I thank my husband for all his support and encouragement.

Pat Blair

October 1997

From the first edition

My especial thanks to: Mr Ainley Wade and Mr Bruce Rhodes of the Royal Pharmaceutical Society of Great Britain; Dr M Keith Thompson, general practitioner; Mr P F Bates, consultant surgeon; and Mr J Pridmore.

May 1985

From the second edition

I am greatly indebted to Ms Anne Prasad of the Royal Pharmaceutical Society of Great Britain; to Mr A C Whitaker for his help with research; and to the Society for permission to use material from the booklet *The Administration and Control of Medicines in Residential Homes*.

July 1991

Section 1
USING MEDICINES MORE EFFECTIVELY

Drugs and Medicines

Whether you buy medicines at the chemist (pharmacist) or supermarket, or whether they are prescribed for you by your doctor, all medicines should be treated with respect. Many years' work have gone into preparing them and great care is taken to ensure that they are as safe as possible – on average it takes 12 years to develop a new medicine to the standard of quality, effectiveness and safety laid down by law. However, there is no such thing as a completely safe medicine. Neither should you expect to receive a medicine every time you visit a doctor. It is not true that there is a 'pill for every ill'. Your doctor's advice and reassurance may be the only medicine you need.

Many medicines have side-effects, or unwanted effects; that is, they act on other parts of your body that are not in need of treatment. For example, certain medicines used to treat infections may also give you diarrhoea or a rash. Side-effects are explained in more detail in the following pages. If you experience any side-effects with your medicine, tell your doctor, nurse or pharmacist so that he or she can help you decide if you should continue taking it. Elderly people are often more sensitive to the effects of medicines, and these effects may also be increased or altered when more than one medicine is taken (see 'The effects of age', p 7).

Because medicines have different effects on different people, you should never give a friend the medicine you take, just because it works for you. Some people may be allergic (over-sensitive) to some medicines: for example, allergy to penicillin and penicillin-like antibiotics is not unusual (see: Your Defence Systems, p 127).

It is equally important when you are prescribed medicines by the doctor that you follow the directions given and finish the course. Do not stop taking the medication just because you feel better. Although pain and discomfort may disappear quickly, drugs need time to do their job properly.

If you have any doubts about what you are taking, consult your doctor or pharmacist. That way both of you will be able to decide what is right for you and how best you remain as healthy as possible. That is why the medicines are used in the first place.

What is a drug?

Basically a drug is anything you take that changes the way your body normally functions. The caffeine in tea and coffee is a drug. So is the alcohol in beer, wine and spirits. The nicotine in tobacco is a drug.

Therapeutic (healing) drugs are used in medicines to restore health. Homoeopathic medicines are therapeutic drugs. Herbal remedies and so-called 'natural' medicines are also drugs. 'Street drugs' – such as heroin, cocaine, cannabis (marijuana), ecstasy – are bought and sold illegally.

Medicines are drugs that are used to keep people healthy or to restore them to health. They divide into four broad groups:

1 Some medicines can be obtained only on a doctor's prescription, which is then dispensed (prepared) by a pharmacist (chemist). These are known as 'prescription-only medicines' (POM).
2 Others – called 'over-the-counter' (OTC) medicines – can be bought without a prescription, but may only be obtained from a pharmacy when a qualified pharmacist is in the shop. They may also be known as pharmacy-only (P) medicines.
3 There are also over-the-counter medicines that can be bought from a chemist, supermarket, corner shop or some health food shops. These are known as general sale list (GSL) medicines.
4 Controlled drugs (CDs) are preparations controlled under the Misuse of Drugs Act. They are available only on a doctor's handwritten prescription. They include most barbiturates, and preparations containing such substances as morphine.

Types of medicine

Medicines often come as tablets, capsules, caplets and powders. As liquids, they can be a mixture or a linctus. Medicines can be inhaled (breathed in) or can come in sprays. They may also be applied as lotions, ointments, creams or gels. They can be given by injection. Some tablets and capsules may have to be swallowed whole; others may have to be crushed. Or they may be placed under your tongue (sublingual) and allowed to dissolve slowly. In addition, tablets and capsules may come in different shapes, sizes and colours.

There are medicines that come in the form of suppositories; these are inserted gently into the rectum through the anus, the hole in your bottom where the waste (stools) comes out. There are also drugs that are contained on patches, similar to sticking plasters, which are placed on the skin. The medicine then passes through the skin into the blood at a regular rate.

Medicine dose and strength

A **dose** of medicine is the amount taken at one time. The **strength** refers to the amount of a particular substance that the medicine contains.

Never take a bigger dose of medicine than you need. If it is a prescribed medicine, your doctor will tell you how much to take, and the instructions should be on the label. If you have bought the medicine at a pharmacy, never take more than the maximum dose marked on the container. It is important to follow the directions.

You should also be aware of the strength of the medication you take. Some medicines are available in one strength only. Others have different strengths. For example, atenolol tablets 100mg are stronger than atenolol tablets 50mg; or aspirin may be in 75mg, 100mg or 300mg strengths. It is the same with medicines you buy. Some medicines have the strength marked with a percentage sign (%), showing how much of the main drug the medicine contains. (In addition, manufacturers' containers and patient information leaflets may list the drug ingredients, with quantities.)

By knowing the strength of your medicine, you can ensure that, each time a prescription is renewed, you are receiving the correct substance. Similarly, if you lose your medicines on holiday, by knowing the strength you will help a doctor or pharmacist to give you the correct replacement. A useful way of keeping track of the details about your medicines is to follow a simple chart like those on pages 15 and 16.

*B*rands of medicine

Medicines can have two names: a 'generic' name and a brand name. The generic name, also known as the 'approved' name, is the descriptive name approved by government agencies. The brand name is given to the medicine by its manufacturer.

In the past, the generic name has come from a list of British Approved Names: it sometimes differed from the name by which the medicine was known abroad. With effect from 1998, however, instead of the British Approved Name, we use the recommended International Nonproprietary Name (INN), where there is one. In the case of a few medicines, this has meant a slight change of name: for example, what was called 'lignocaine' is now 'lidocaine', what was 'oestradiol' is now 'estradiol', and 'phenobarbitone' is now 'phenobarbital'. Some medicine labels and patient information sheets may carry both the British Approved Name and the recommended International Nonproprietary Name. The medicine, however, remains the same.

With both branded and generic products, the same type of medicine may be dispensed as tablets of different shapes, colours, sizes and names, depending on their manufacturer. For example, Amfipen and Penbritin (brand names) are different manufacturers' names for ampicillin (generic name). The brand name and the generic name will both appear somewhere on the medicine container label. Some doctors write the brand name on the prescription form (in which case the pharmacist must supply *only* that particular version). Others write the generic name. Whichever is used, you will be getting the medication you need.

The doctor may write the approved (generic) name on the prescription form, and the pharmacist may then supply a branded variety. This practice occurs because the pharmacist usually has to supply the cheapest form of the prescribed medication, to keep down costs to the National Health Service (NHS). In such cases, you may sometimes receive a different colour, shape or size of tablet than the one you have become used to. If you are unsure about this, check with the pharmacist that it is your usual medication. And if the new medicine has side-effects that you have never had before, tell your doctor.

Paying for medicines

Most prescribed medicines are free to men and women aged 60 or over. However, not all medicines are available on NHS prescription. Government guidelines, issued to doctors and pharmacists, list the medicines that can, and cannot, be supplied on NHS prescription. These guidelines are known as the 'limited list'. The list was produced to save money on the cost of drugs to the NHS and is updated from time to time.

This does mean, however, that some medicines you previously received may no longer be available on free prescription. In such cases, your doctor may decide on another, equally effective medicine that is available on an NHS prescription. If this happens, you should check for side-effects (see below) and, if you have any, report them to your doctor.

Alternatively, you may be offered the option of paying for a particular drug or brand of medicine on a private prescription. It is an option that you are perfectly entitled to refuse. Remember, the price you would be paying is the full cost of the medicine, not just the general prescription charge; and medicines can be very expensive. In the case of private prescriptions there may also be a dispensing charge added by the pharmacist.

Some prescribed medicines, including those available on NHS prescription, can also be bought 'over the counter'. In some instances this may cost less than any prescription charge. If you are not entitled to a free prescription, it may be worth asking the doctor or the pharmacist which is the cheaper option.

Side-effects, or unwanted effects

When a drug goes into your bloodstream it is carried round to many parts of your body and can have effects other than those you and your doctor are seeking. These are what are known as side-effects, or unwanted effects. When you are prescribed a medicine, make sure you know what effects you can expect from it. Most doctors are happy to give you that advice.

Among some side-effects are: feeling faint or dizzy; becoming confused; feeling sick; developing rashes or a dry mouth; having blurred vision. Diarrhoea, constipation and a thumping heart are some other side-effects mentioned in the book. Similarly, some medicines can affect your sex drive or cause impotence. Not everyone experiences such effects, but if you do, you should let your doctor know about them.

Some side-effects can be prevented by changing the dosage or the timing, or by changing to another medicine. Some may be due to the way you are taking your medicine: you may be taking too much, too often; or you may be taking too little and not often enough. If you have to report side-effects, tell your doctor how often and how much medicine you have been taking. He or she can then help you decide if the medicine is right for you. Some side-effects cannot be helped.

The effects of age

As you grow older, your body handles drugs differently. Drugs are processed and eliminated from your system more slowly. As a result, higher amounts of the medicines you take remain in your body for longer periods than would be the case in someone younger. With age, you can become more sensitive to drugs and that can lead to you experiencing side-effects. These effects can become magnified if you are also frail, debilitated or acutely ill.

Drug interaction

Sometimes if you take two or more types of drug they can act against each other in your body. The action of one drug may be increased.

Or it may be reduced. Doctors and pharmacists are aware of these effects. They can, however, advise you only if you keep them informed about the medicines you take. You should tell your doctor if, in addition to prescribed medicines, you are taking ones that you have bought yourself.

Equally, you should ask the pharmacist's advice if you plan to buy medicines in addition to those you already take, whether you have bought them yourself or have been prescribed them by your doctor. This will also help prevent you taking an accidental overdose of some substances. An overdose of paracetamol, for example, is dangerous, and can be fatal. A useful painkiller, it is also included in some cold remedies. Although 'contains paracetamol' is often marked clearly on the cold remedy label, some people have also treated themselves with tablets, and other paracetamol-containing remedies, with disastrous consequences.

Because of the interaction of some drugs with certain foods, drinks or alcohol, you may be advised to avoid taking a particular medicine near the time you have a specific food or drink. Or you may be advised not to take certain food, or alcohol, at all while you are on that medication.

*P*atient information leaflets

– Most medicines contain a 'patient information leaflet' in their packaging. This is intended by the manufacturers to give you fuller details about the medicine, what it contains, what it is for, the recommended dose, side-effects, what precautions to take, and how to store it. You should read such leaflets carefully and not dispose of them until you have finished with the medicine.

Sometimes the dose recommended on the information leaflet may be different from the dose prescribed for you by your doctor. If that is the case, check with your doctor that you are taking the correct dose intended for you.

Getting Advice

You and the doctor

You and the doctor are a partnership. You provide basic information about your health that the doctor needs; the doctor provides advice, discusses the options available, and may prescribe medication. When you obtain a prescription and follow the instructions for taking the medicine, you should also note any results from taking it and tell the doctor of any untoward effects. It is important to maintain this partnership with the doctor, whether you see him or her at your home, at the surgery, or in a clinic or hospital.

Sometimes, instead of your usual doctor, you may see a locum, or a deputising doctor. You should still ask that doctor the questions that are listed below. If you are being visited at home, a deputising doctor may give you a letter; and it is in your own interest to make sure your own doctor receives the letter.

Before seeing the doctor

Before you visit the doctor, or before the doctor calls to see you, prepare a list of things to tell the doctor and questions you want to ask. If you are unable to do this, ask a friend or relative.

Among the things you should put on your list are:

1 The medicines you are taking. Include those that you have bought over the counter as well as those that have been prescribed for you. Some you may take regularly, others you may use only occasionally. Tell your doctor about *all* of them. The doctor needs to know about the medicines you take so that he or she does not

duplicate them or prescribe medicines that will cause a bad reaction when taken together.

2 Which medicines, if any, do not agree with you.
3 A note of any allergies you may have.

Things to ask the doctor

If your doctor prescribes a medicine, make sure that you have some facts about each drug you are given. Write these down, or ask the doctor to do so. Do not rely on your memory; many people forget exactly what has been said. If your doctor tells you to use your medicine 'as required', ask what that means.

Facts you should know:

1 The name of the medicine.
2 What it is for.
3 If there are any foods, drinks or other medicines you should avoid while taking the new medicine.
4 When you should take the medicine.
5 How much you should take at a time.
6 How long you should continue taking it.
7 What you should do if you miss taking a dose.
8 If you will need another prescription; if so, when?
9 Are there any side-effects?
10 Are there things you should not do while taking the medicine, such as driving a car or operating machinery?

You and the pharmacist (chemist)

The pharmacist or chemist is an expert on drugs and their effects. He or she may work in the hospital pharmacy, in a health centre, or in a pharmacy in the high street or shopping centre. It is preferable to get to know your pharmacist by name, especially if you need medication regularly. It can also be helpful to register with one pharmacy, whether you are buying medicines or having prescriptions prepared. Many pharmacies now keep medicine records for their regular customers; in that way they can help you keep track of what you are taking.

Choosing your pharmacy (chemist's shop)

Select your pharmacy with care. Take into account how easy it is for you to reach. Although a number of shops sell non-prescription medicines, a pharmacy must by law have a qualified pharmacist to dispense medicines and give advice. A shop in which there is a qualified pharmacist usually displays a sticker, card or sign that has a green cross and the word 'pharmacy' written on it. It looks like this:

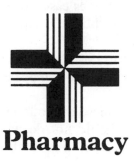

Pharmacy

Things to ask the pharmacist

Whether you are buying over-the-counter medicines or obtaining a prescription, your pharmacist can give you information about the drugs and their effect(s). If you are already taking medicines, take a list of them with you to show the pharmacist. If you are also using herbal remedies, or supplements from a health-food shop, include these on your list. The pharmacist can then advise you whether the medicine you propose to buy will interfere with anything you are already taking. In many cases, warnings will be printed on the medicine container's label. Most medicines now have, in their container, a leaflet that gives further information about them. Or the pharmacist may give you a leaflet containing advice about the medicine and what, if anything, to avoid. You should read any such leaflets carefully.

Your pharmacist can give you information, or extra information, about the following:

1 Proper times to take medicines.
2 Whether the medicine has an expiry date.
3 Side-effects of over-the-counter and prescription medicines.
4 Which over-the-counter medicines will be most suitable for you and the ailment you wish to treat.
5 Whether the over-the-counter medicines, or those prescribed for you, will interfere with anything you are already taking, or if you should avoid certain foods or drinks.
6 How to open medicine containers. Your pharmacist will replace child-resistant caps with ones easier to remove if you ask. If you have difficulty opening 'blister packs', you should discuss this with the pharmacist.
7 Where you should store your medicines. A bathroom cabinet, where the air is damp and warm, may be exactly the wrong place to keep it.
8 What to do with medicines you no longer take.
9 Are there things you should not do while taking the medicine, such as driving a car or operating machinery?
10 If your medicine is in liquid form, ask for the correct size of measure and check how much you need to take each time.

You and the nurse

You may be in regular contact with a nurse. Some work at the doctor's surgery, where they are known as practice nurses. (They should not be confused with the doctor's receptionist, who may or may not be a nurse.) Some nurses work in clinics. Others may call regularly to see you at your home. These may be community or district nurses, or other nurses and their helpers working in the nursing team. Or they may be health visitors, nurses who are specially trained to help prevent you from becoming ill.

Although most nurses themselves are not experts in drugs and their effects, they are trained to recognise any problems you may have with your medicines. Nurses can find out the answers to any questions you may have about the medicines you use. They can also help you work out a system for taking your medicines if you have to do so regularly. They can show you how to open containers and advise you how to store medicines at home. If you have problems with opening blister packs, the nurse can help you. There are also some medicines and special dressings that they may be able to order for you.

If you have any difficulties with the medicines you take, tell the nurse. If you know he or she is going to call, make a list of the questions you wish to have answered.

Taking Your Medicine

To get the most benefit from the medicines your doctor prescribes or from those you buy, and to reduce any risks, you must take them according to the directions. This becomes more difficult if you have more than one type of medicine to take. It is especially so if the medicines have to be taken at different times. You may find it useful to organise a system for taking your drugs – or get someone to help you do so.

Make sure that the system you choose works for you. There is no point in choosing one that you find too complicated. Below are four examples of systems.

A simple chart

On a simple chart you can list the name of the drug and its strength; what it is for; what shape and colour it is; how often it should be taken and when (before meals, during or after meals); how it should be taken (with water, mixed in water, swallowed whole, placed under your tongue or chewed). You should note whether it makes you feel sleepy or any other effects you may expect; whether there are any foods, drinks or other medicines you must avoid while you are taking it. Put down the time of day when it should be taken, such as 8.00am, 2.00pm and 8.00pm, or 'first thing in the morning', 'last thing at night'.

Keep the chart near where you keep your medicines. It should be kept up to date, as the shape and size of medicines can change with each prescription if a different brand is supplied by the pharmacist. On the next page is an example of a simple chart for you to copy.

Name of drug Strength What it's for	Colour/ shape	Directions Things to avoid	Times

A weekly checking chart

This type of chart can be used both for listing your medicines and for checking that you have taken them. It could be written out on a postcard for carrying about when you are away from home. Or it can be attached to a piece of card and hung on the wall near your medicines. Keep a pen or pencil beside it.

Overleaf is an example of a weekly checking chart. It shows how to fill it in with the times you take your medicines. From it you will see that the patient takes drug 'A' at 8.00am, 1.00pm and 7.00pm every day. Drug 'B' is taken once a day, at 8.00am. The correct time is ticked for each drug when it has been taken. The imaginary patient on this chart has taken all of Sunday's medicines. He has taken Monday's only up to 1.00pm.

A daily container

If you take the same medicines every day, and can tell which medicine is which, you may prefer to use a daily container. This could be a pill-box, an eggcup or a plastic box; or you could buy a special container. Each morning, you place all the tablets for that day into the container. Then at any time of the day you can see how many tablets you have taken and how many are left to take. That way you should

1 Name of drug / 2 What it's for / 3 Colour/shape / 4 Directions	SUN	MON	TUE	WED	THU	FRI	SAT
1 Drug 'A' 2 Blood Pressure 3 White Tablets 4 3 Times Daily	8.00 / 1.00 / 7.00	8.00 / 1.00 / 7.00	8.00 / 1.00 / 7.00	8.00 / 1.00 / 7.00	8.00 / 1.00 / 7.00	8.00 / 1.00 / 7.00	8.00 / 1.00 / 7.00
1 Drug 'B' 2 Heart 3 Pink Capsules 4 One in morning	8.00	8.30	8.30	8.30	8.00	8.00	8.00

never take more than prescribed, nor will you take too few. You could get confused by this system, though, if two or more of the tablets are similar in size and shape.

A weekly container

If you have to take some tablets every day, but others only once or twice a week, a container with more compartments may suit you. It may also be useful if you have some tablets that look similar. There are a number of containers you can buy. Your doctor, pharmacist or nurse may be able to help you choose one if you think you would like to use a weekly container. Some of them can be awkward for arthritic hands, so before buying, check that you can open the container.

Important points about containers

Not all medicines are suitable for transfer to a container. Some tablets must be kept in the bottles, boxes or packs in which they are supplied. Check whether it is all right to put your tablets in your chosen container.

Remember If children are likely to visit, you should not put containers where they can reach them. All medicines – including herbal remedies – should be kept out of children's way, but special containers are often easier to open. Never put sweets in containers that are like pill-boxes – and vice versa.

Many tablets are supplied in blister packs or in containers that are deliberately made more difficult for young children to open. These are called child-resistant containers, of which there are a number of types. When you receive your medication, you should ask for a leaflet explaining how to open and close the containers, or get the pharmacist to show you.

Unfortunately, containers that are difficult for children to open are also sometimes difficult for older people to manage. In that case you should ask for an ordinary container. Tell the pharmacist if you have problems opening blister packs.

*H*ospital – outpatients and day surgery

If you attend hospital as an outpatient, you may be treated with a medicine that could have side-effects. Before you leave the hospital, ask the doctor or nurse if there are any side-effects that you should know about. This is especially important if you have been given medicines that may make you drowsy, including an anaesthetic, in which case you should not drive a car or operate machinery.

Many people now have operations as day surgery: they go into hospital in the morning, have their operation and then leave in the evening. Check with the doctor or nurse whether there are likely to be any side-effects from medicines you have been given before, during or after the operation.

*R*epeat prescriptions

You may be receiving long-term medication, for diabetes or blood pressure problems for example. If you need a regular supply of medicine, your doctor may give you a card that you take back to the surgery every time you need more medication. The card will contain details of the medicine or medicines you need and will be used at your doctor's surgery to write a further prescription. You should hand both the prescription and the card to your pharmacist, so that the pharmacist can check that the details are correct.

It is important that you see your doctor in person at regular intervals, if you are receiving medicines through this system of repeat prescriptions. How often may depend on your age and your ailment. In any event, you should not leave it longer than three months, unless you have agreed a different timetable with your doctor. However, if there is a change in your condition, do not wait until your next agreed visit is due. Instead, you should make an appointment to see your doctor in the normal way.

Withdrawn drugs

From time to time, a government committee issues instructions to doctors not to prescribe any more of a certain drug. This may be because new side-effects of the drug have come to light. The committee may then feel that the risks of the drug are greater than the benefits it brings. You may see reports of these cases in your newspaper, or hear them on radio or television. If that happens, it is important that you do **not** stop taking the medicine. Continue with it but make an early appointment to see your doctor. He or she can then advise you what to do. Because the doctor has been given more detailed information about why the drug is being withdrawn, he or she may consider that it is all right for you to continue taking it. Alternatively, something else may be prescribed.

The same applies if you hear that a drug has been 'suspended'. That means that the government committee is being cautious until it has more information from doctors and manufacturers. Do not stop taking it – see your doctor first.

Difficulties in getting medicine you need

Some medicines are no longer available on NHS prescription generally (see 'Paying for medicines', p 6), but you should not be denied prescribable medicines merely because of your age. Sometimes there is a good reason: some medicines can be unsafe for older people's use, or the safety of newer medicines may not yet have been established in older people (see 'The effects of age', p 7). However, you should not be denied essential medicine, including expensive medication, on the basis of its cost. If you have difficulty in getting the medicine you need, you should contact your local health authority, community health council, an Age Concern or similar group, or an appropriate self-help group (see: Useful Addresses, p 136)

Problems in taking medicine

It is helpful to find out beforehand what to do if there is a mishap when you are taking prescribed medicines. Such mishaps can include: forgetting to take a dose; taking a dose twice; being sick just after taking your medicine; having diarrhoea just after using a suppository. Check beforehand with your doctor, just in case. Do not assume that, because you have missed one dose, you can take twice as much next time.

Some drugs – for example, steroids – must never be stopped, except under a doctor's supervision. This is because the effects of suddenly stopping the medication could be harmful and even dangerous (see also the section on corticosteroids in: Your Glandular System). If you are taking such drugs, always carry with you the special card given to you by your doctor or pharmacist. Then, if you have an accident, the people who help you will know that the drug you are taking must be continued.

At home, you should keep your doctor's telephone number near your telephone; when you are away from home, take the number with you.

Storing medicines

Medicines can be dangerous. If used wrongly or stored carelessly they can be harmful to you, young children, your family and pets.

Medicines, like foods, do not last for ever. Some become ineffective sooner than others. Do not keep medicines past their expiry date, which may be printed on the label or somewhere on the container. Many medicines should be kept in a cool, dry place, whereas others have to be kept away from the light. Check the label for any special instructions concerning your medicine. That applies equally to the medicines you have bought over the counter and those that have been prescribed for you.

Do not keep medicines just in case the ailment comes back. Even if you get symptoms that you have had before, you might not have the same ailment, or your condition may have changed and you may need a different drug. A third possibility is that the medicine may be too old to use safely. It is always better to check with your doctor.

Disposing of unwanted medicines

If you have medicines you no longer use, when you next see your doctor, nurse or pharmacist, ask how to dispose of the medicines. Do not put them in your dustbin, in case they are accidentally picked up by children or by pets. Pharmacists will dispose of unwanted medicines for you.

Sharing medicines

Never share with a friend medicines that have been prescribed for you. And do not use someone else's prescribed medicine. Both can be dangerous. When prescribing, your doctor takes into account all your symptoms, how drugs will act on them and whether you are taking other medicines. People with a similar ailment to yours may be prescribed different medicines because of the different ways drugs react in different people, or because they are already taking other medication.

The dangers of swapping medicines apply not only to prescribed medicines. The same principles apply to those you buy at a chemist's or supermarket. The best thing you can do for a friend is to encourage him or her to ask a pharmacist or a doctor for advice.

Living in country areas

If you live in the country, or in what – for official NHS purposes – is designated a rural area, there may be special arrangements available to help you get your prescriptions filled. There are a number of different systems, and not every system is used in every area. For example, the pharmacist may arrange to have your prescription delivered to you; the post van may take your prescription forms and deliver the medicine a day or two later; voluntary organisations may run a local scheme.

In some cases, your doctor may be allowed to dispense your prescription. That depends on the health authority responsible for medical, pharmacy, dental and opticians' services in your area. The health authority's address will be in your telephone directory, or you can get it from your doctor, or from the Health Information Service on its free helpline (Tel: 0800 66 55 44). The health authority should be able to advise you which local schemes can help you obtain your prescription. The community health council or your local Age Concern group may also help. Their addresses should be in your telephone directory.

Going on holiday

Going on holiday should not pose any problems but there are some sensible precautions to take. Don't take just enough medicines for the time you are going to be away. Pack a few days' extra supply in case there are delays of buses, trains or planes. Remember to take your medicine chart (plus pen or pencil). Make sure you have your doctor's address and telephone number. Also take with you a note of the name of your medicine – the generic name as well as the brand name – and the strength. Carry your medicines in your hand luggage if you are flying – just in case your baggage goes astray.

Replacing lost medicines

If you lose your medicines while you are on holiday do not despair. If you are in the United Kingdom but cannot get a local doctor, go to a pharmacy. If you can convince the pharmacist that you know the correct medicine you need, the pharmacist may sell you enough to keep you going until you see a local doctor. Remember that the pharmacist will not be able to supply the medicine free; you will have to pay the full price, which can be expensive. And the maximum the pharmacist can sell you is five days' supply.

If you are abroad and lose your medicine, it is even more important that you know what it is, rather than just the brand name. The same drug may be sold under a different brand name overseas. To help

yourself, the doctor and the pharmacist – at home or abroad – you
need to 'know your medicines'.

Living in a residential home

Medicines are the property of the resident for whom they are prescribed. They should not be given to anyone else. If you live in a
residential home and wish to look after your own medication, you
should have a lockable cupboard in which you can keep all your
medicines.

If a resident is not able to look after his or her own medication, the
medicine should be kept in the container in which it is supplied and
the resident's name written clearly on it. An individual's medicines
should not be mixed in a single container with his or her previous
medicine or with those prescribed for other people, even if the medicines seem to be the same. That is the way errors occur. Similar
medicines may actually come from different batches, their expiry
dates may differ or they may be of different strengths. All medicines
should be locked away safely.

If a resident leaves the home or transfers to another home, personal
medicines should be handed back to him or her, or destroyed – after
checking with his or her doctor.

Keeping records in residential homes

There should be three types of record in residential homes: a central
register, or medicines book, to record all medicines that come into
the home; an individual record for each resident, recording their
medication and such things as allergies; an administration record, on
which is recorded all the medicines they have taken. The person in
charge of the home should ensure that the records are kept and
retained for a minimum of three years after the death of a resident.

Procedures for administering medicines in homes

Do not transfer medicines to egg-cups or individual pots ready to give out to residents; that can lead to error, as it means the medicines are separated from the instructions on the container label written by the pharmacist. There are six steps to follow if residents are given medicine by home care staff. They apply whether they are prescribed medicines or over-the-counter remedies. Care staff should be trained in this procedure, which should also be followed when preparing a daily or weekly container for an individual resident to use.

1 Check the identity of the resident.
2 Look at the resident's record card and check the person's name and the dose instructions, looking particularly to see if there have been any recent changes in his or her medication and that it has not already been given.
3 Identify the resident's medicine container and check that its label matches the record card.
4 Give the medicine to the resident.
5 Note on the record card that the medicine has been given.
6 Record if the resident did not take the medicine, and say why. When a medicine has been taken from its container and not taken by the resident, the medicine should not be returned to the container but should be destroyed by the member of staff who is responsible for medicines in the home.

Disposing of medicines in homes

Medicines to be destroyed should be returned to the pharmacist who supplied them, or destroyed under his or her supervision. Medicines should be disposed of safely when their expiry date is reached or if any is left when the course of treatment is completed or changed. Special care should be taken with eye ointments, as these generally have short expiry dates after they have been opened. If the resident for whom medicines are prescribed dies, the medicines should be kept for seven days after the death, in case they are wanted by the coroner's office. When medicines are destroyed, this should be noted on the record card, and should be witnessed.

Section 2
MEDICINES AND YOUR BODY SYSTEMS

Your Digestive System

A little of what you fancy does you good, so the old song goes. But too much of what you fancy has the opposite effect. Never was it more true than in the case of food and digestion. Careful eating, and eating the foods that are good for you, will go a long way to keeping your digestive system in order. Ailments such as wind, feeling sick, indigestion or ulcers are made worse by drinking too much alcohol and by smoking.

The digestive system is a very effective food processor involving many muscles and organs, from top to bottom. Even before food enters your mouth, the food processor starts to work, at the sight, smell or even the thought of food. In the mouth, saliva (mouth watering) is a digestive juice that is produced.

Saliva moistens the food and mixes with it to start to break it down into the substances that the body can take in. Chewing is needed for the saliva to mix with the food, making the mixture easier to swallow. The tongue is important in this procedure of guiding the food around. The taste buds are in the tongue.

Swallowing, a squeezing action of throat muscles, pushes the food over the throat and down the oesophagus (gullet) into the stomach. This squeezing action, called peristalsis, happens throughout the digestive system to push food and food products through the body.

The stomach, which contains juices to help digest the food further, acts as a store or reservoir. It also churns the food, mixing it more thoroughly with the gastric (stomach) juices. It releases small amounts of the mixture at intervals into the intestines (guts, bowel) where more juices are added. There the body absorbs food substances when they have been broken down into simple chemical forms. The rate at which the stomach releases the food mixture depends on the rate at which you eat, the type of food eaten and even the mood you are in when you eat it.

A number of glands are involved at various stages of digestion. Apart from the salivary glands, there are others in the stomach, pancreas and liver. The liver also manufactures bile, which is then stored in the gall-bladder until it is needed.

The liver is an important organ that has a variety of functions. During digestion it acts as a storage vessel for the body's basic fuel, glucose, a sugar derived from carbohydrates. Glucose is converted into glycogen for storage. The liver reconverts it to glucose and releases it, as needed, to supply the blood with a steady level of sugar. Liver cells can make glucose out of protein and fats. They are able to convert excess sugar into fat and send it for storage in other parts of your body. The liver also makes essential proteins and stocks certain vitamins until they are needed by other organs. It checks the protein products that have passed through the digestive system, rejecting those the body cannot use, which are taken away by the kidney and the bowel. In addition, the liver filters and destroys bacteria and neutralises some poisons. (For more on the liver and pancreas, see: Your Glandular System.)

The intestines consist of the small and large intestines. The small intestine is where most of the food digestion takes place. The first part, called the duodenum, leads directly from the stomach. The small intestine (which is about 6.7 metres (22 feet) long) leads into the large intestine. That consists of parts called the caecum, the colon and the rectum. Your appendix is attached to the caecum. The small intestine extracts the nutrients the body needs. The large intestine extracts water that the body needs to save; its last part is the rectum, and the indigestible matter (stools, faeces, motions) eventually leaves the body through the anus (the hole in the bottom). How often people get rid of the waste matter varies. Most people have a bowel movement at least every day, but your normal pattern may be different.

Common ailments

As you grow older, you may produce less saliva and so your mouth feels drier when you eat. That makes chewing even more important. Badly fitted false teeth will stop you chewing properly and can cause you to swallow more air, giving you flatulence (wind). Your senses of taste and smell may be reduced. An inflamed tongue can indicate to your doctor a number of disorders, including deficiencies in your diet.

Sore throats, which may be a sign of other illnesses, may also be due to infection and should be checked. A dry mouth and throat will happen if you are upset, perhaps worried or depressed – but that can happen at any age. Difficulties in swallowing should be reported to your doctor, especially if they persist.

The oesophagus (gullet) can become inflamed due to reflux (food and gastric juice coming back up, a feeling of being sick). The acid effects of this can also cause pain and bleeding. Reflux, which should be checked with your doctor, can be due to a number of causes, including hiatus hernia, when part of the stomach slips upwards through the diaphragm, a thin flat muscle.

The stomach walls can be less efficient in older people. Gastric (stomach) acids, peptic and other juices may be produced more slowly and in smaller amounts, leading to food digestion taking longer. You may therefore not feel as hungry as quickly as you did when you were younger, although a serious loss of appetite should be discussed with your doctor as it can be a sign of illness. However, because the stomach does its work more slowly, the food mixture will also be released more slowly from it.

Ulcers in the stomach (gastric ulcers) and in the duodenum (duodenal ulcers) affect people of many ages, but older people especially. Some ulcers may be linked to infection by a bacterium, *Helicobacter pylori* (*H pylori*). The term 'peptic ulcers' covers both types of ulcer. Gastritis is inflammation of the stomach.

Disease of the liver, inflammation of the gall-bladder or gall-stones can interfere with the flow of bile into the duodenum. Many older people suffer from gall-stones that form in the gall-bladder.

Sometimes a stone escapes and blocks the duct, or tube, through which the bile travels to the intestine; this can be painful. Pancreatitis, inflammation of the pancreas, happens for a number of reasons and is associated with gall-bladder problems. It can also be due to alcohol abuse.

Stomach cramps, or spasms, may affect various parts of the intestine. Spasms may be due to muscles in the intestine's walls squeezing too hard and can lead to constipation – difficulty in passing hard, dry stools – or to diarrhoea – passing watery stools. (For trouble with your waterworks, see: Your Kidneys and 'Waterworks'.)

Spasms may also be caused by diverticulitis, an inflammation or soreness in small pockets of the bowel. Irritable bowel syndrome is inflammation of the colon and it, too, can cause spasms, stomach pains, diarrhoea and/or constipation, or flatulence (wind). Colitis, which can affect the colon and rectum, is another ailment that has effects similar to those of irritable bowel syndrome.

Crohn's disease, an ailment in which parts of the intestine become inflamed and thickened, can cause pain, diarrhoea or an inability to absorb some foods.

Problems with emptying the bowel may occur, although this is not necessarily due to age. If there is any change in the frequency or pattern of times you normally pass stools, or if there is blood in your stools, you should tell your doctor, as that can be a sign of illness. Constipation does not depend on how often you go to the toilet but on how hard it is to go. Your diet may be at fault – for example, you may not be taking enough roughage or fluid. Constipation could also be a side-effect of drugs you are taking, or you may not be getting enough exercise. Incontinence (not being able to control your bowel) may have similar causes. (See also bladder problems on p 85.)

Diarrhoea is a frequent emptying of the bowel, or the passing of unusually loose or watery stools. If it is serious, or goes on longer than 12 hours, you should call your doctor, because loss of fluid or salts from your body can cause problems in itself. Diarrhoea can be due to infection, or it may be a side-effect of some medicines, or a symptom of another bowel ailment.

Haemorrhoids (piles) are swollen veins in the rectum (back passage) and can be caused by, among other things, straining to pass hard, dry stools. These in turn may be due to a lack of fibre in your diet. (See also 'Local anaesthetic drugs' in: Your Skin, p 112.)

What medicines do

All but a few medicines taken by mouth go through the digestive system in the same way as food. Depending on the ingredients from which they are made, they act on the digestive system in various ways, as food itself does. Check with the pharmacist that new medicines will not interfere with any you already take.

Antacids

Antacids are often taken to relieve the discomfort of ulcers or indigestion (dyspepsia, heartburn, upset stomach). They act by neutralising or diluting the stomach acids and this helps stop the pain. The various antacids contain different ingredients and not all may be suitable for every person. Depending on what the antacids are made from, they may cause some substances to be absorbed more quickly by your body, and others to be absorbed more slowly. People who have problems with their heart or their kidneys or who have liver disease should also take advice before using antacids. Some have a laxative effect, but others may make you constipated. Some mixtures may cause your body to retain fluid, and are not suitable if you take diuretics or are on a low-salt diet. For all these reasons, if you decide to buy antacids, ask the pharmacist if they are suitable for you. Liquid antacids are more effective but tablets may be more convenient.

If your doctor plans to give you medication, tell him or her what you have been taking for your indigestion. You should not take antacids regularly without checking with your doctor, in person. Common antacids include the following.

Aluminium-containing antacids

These may cause constipation. They may affect how your body absorbs some antibiotics and iron. Antacids of this type include:

Actal, Alu-Cap, Aludrox gel/liquid, Asilone tablets, etc.

ALUMINIUM AND MAGNESIUM ANTACIDS

These are less likely to cause constipation or diarrhoea but may affect how your body absorbs some antibiotics. They should not be used by people with kidney problems. Antacids of this type include: *Actonorm gel, Altacite, Aludrox Tablets, Asilone Liquid, Boots Double Action Indigestion, Dijex, Entrotabs, Gastrocote, Gaviscon, Gelusil, Maalox, Mucogel, Sovol.*

CALCIUM-CONTAINING ANTACIDS

These should not be taken for long periods without seeking advice. Antacids of this type include: *Andrews Antacid, Barum Antacid, BiSoDol tablets, Boots Indigestion Tablets, De Witt's tablets, Opas, Rennie Gold, Setlers, Tums,* etc.

MAGNESIUM-CONTAINING ANTACIDS

Antacids such as these may cause you to pass looser stools than you usually do. Different magnesium mixtures include: magnesium carbonate, magnesium hydroxide and magnesium trisilicate. They should not be used by people with kidney problems. Antacids of this type include: *Andrews Antacid, Bismag, BiSoDol, Boots Indigestion Tablets, De Witt's tablets, Milk of Magnesia,* etc.

SODIUM BICARBONATE ANTACIDS

Burping may be caused by these. They may contain a high dose of sodium and should be avoided by people who need to take diuretics or who have been told to keep their salt intake down. It is important to realise that, although Alka-Seltzer contains sodium bicarbonate, and people use it as an antacid, its main ingredient is aspirin, which can irritate the stomach. Remedies containing aspirin should be avoided if you have peptic ulcers, stomach upsets, asthma or if you are taking medicines for blood disorders. Antacids containing sodium bicarbonate include: *BiSoDol, Boots Headache and Indigestion Relief* (contains paracetamol), *De Witt's powder, Gaviscon, Opas, Resolve, Soda mint tablets,* etc.

Laxatives

Laxatives are drugs that are generally used to treat constipation. They may be taken as tablets, granules or liquid, or as suppositories which are inserted in the rectum (by pushing them gently up your bottom). If your doctor, nurse or pharmacist gives you suppositories, which to some people may seem like very large tablets, you should ask how to use them.

Laxatives should not be taken as a habit. Occasional use may be all right but if you feel you need to take them often, check with your doctor. They often consist of a mixture of ingredients and can be broadly divided into the following four main groups.

BULK-FORMING LAXATIVES

These increase the amount of the stools (motions, faeces, waste matter), which in turn encourages the muscle action of the bowel (peristalsis). It is essential that you drink plenty of fluid with this type of laxative, and that you stop taking it if it fails to work within a few days. It may give you wind. You should not take it just before bedtime. Laxatives of this type include: *bran preparations, Celevac, Fybogel, Isogel, ispaghula husk, Manevac, Normacol, Regulan.*

STIMULANT LAXATIVES

By stimulating the lining of the bowel, these increase the action of the bowel muscles. They may cause discomfort or spasms. Some preparations may colour your urine (water) red. Laxatives of this type include: *bisacodyl, cascara, castor oil, Codalax, dantron [danthron], Dulco-lax, Ex-lax, glycerol, Manevac, Normax, senna, Senokot, syrup of figs.*

SOFTENERS

Such laxatives lubricate and soften the stools, which may then be more easy to pass. If you feel you need them regularly, check first with your doctor. Laxatives of this type include: *Agarol, Dioctyl* (also slightly stimulant), *Normax, liquid paraffin.*

OSMOTIC LAXATIVES

These laxatives cause the bowel to retain water and thus increase the amount of the stools. You should drink plenty of fluid when you take these and should not take them if you are taking diuretic drugs. Laxatives of this type include: *Andrews Liver Salts, Epsom Salts, Milk of Magnesia, Lactugal, lactulose, Laxose, Movicol, Osmolax, Regulose.*

Some other drugs and their brand names

Alverine citrate *Relaxyl, Spasmonal*

If you have irritable bowel syndrome or diverticulitis, this may be used to treat the pain and relax intestinal muscles. Possible side-effects: feeling sick, headache, itching, rash, dizziness, allergy.

Belladonna alkaloids *Aluhyde, Bellocarb, Carbellon*, etc

These act on the nervous system to reduce the movement of muscles in the stomach and the intestines. Their unwanted effects make them unsuitable if you have glaucoma or an enlarged prostate. Possible side-effects: blurred vision, dry mouth, difficulty in passing urine, rapid beating of the heart (palpitations), constipation.

Cimetidine *Algitec, Dyspamet, Tagamet*

As this reduces the stomach's production of acids, it may be used to treat peptic ulcers, reflux and some dyspepsias. You should not take antacids with cimetidine unless your doctor agrees. Possible side-effects: dizziness, skin rash, changed bowel habits, tiredness, impotence.

Dicycloverine hydrochloride [dicyclomine hydrochloride] *Kolanticon, Merbentyl*, etc

This acts on the nervous system to reduce the movement of muscles in the stomach and intestine and may help irritable bowels. Possible side-effects: slightly blurred eyesight, dry mouth, rapid beating of the heart (palpitations), retention of urine (water), constipation.

Lansoprazole *Zoton*

This acts to reduce the stomach's production of acid. You may be prescribed this, perhaps together with an antibiotic, if you suffer from reflux, heartburn or gastric ulcers. Possible side-effects: skin rash, itching, headache, diarrhoea, sickness, constipation, wind, stomach pain, dizziness, blurred eyesight, pains in joints.

Loperamide hydrochloride *Imodium, Arret, etc*

This may be used to treat problems of diarrhoea. It should not be used for longer than three days, unless your doctor tells you otherwise. Possible side-effects: constipation, stomach pains, skin rash.

Mesalazine *Asacol, Pentasa, Salofalk*

This may be used if you have ulcerative colitis. Possible side-effects: feeling sick, diarrhoea, stomach pains. You should tell your doctor if you have fever, unexplained bleeding or bruising, a sore throat or if the medicine makes you feel weak.

Misoprostol *Cytotec*

This reduces the stomach's production of acids. It may be used to prevent peptic ulcers or to help in healing them. You should avoid magnesium-containing antacids if you are taking this medicine. Possible side-effects: diarrhoea, stomach upsets, wind.

Olsalazine *Dipentum*

This may be used if you have ulcerative colitis. Possible side-effects: feeling sick, diarrhoea, headache, stomach cramps, rash. You should tell your doctor if you have fever, unexplained bleeding or bruising, a sore throat or if the medicine makes you feel weak.

Omeprazole *Losec*

This reduces the stomach's production of acid. It may be used for peptic ulcers and reflux. Possible side-effects: feeling sick, changed bowel habits, wind, headache, rashes.

Oral rehydration salts *Dioralyte, Diocalm Replenish, Electrolade, Rehidrat, etc*

These may be used to replace fluid and essential salts lost as a result of mild diarrhoea and/or vomiting. They may contain sodium, potassium, citrate, bicarbonate and glucose. If you have diabetes and take oral hydration salts, you should monitor your blood-sugar levels.

Pancreatin *Nutrizym, Pancrex, etc*

This is used to aid digestion in pancreatic disease. Possible side-effects: skin irritation around the mouth or anus.

Peppermint oil *Colpermin, Mintec*

This relaxes intestinal muscles and may be used for abdominal pain or distension (feeling bloated), especially in irritable bowel syndrome. You should swallow such capsules whole and not chew them, as the oil can irritate your mouth and oesophagus (gullet). Possible side-effects: heartburn.

Propantheline *Pro-Banthine*

This acts on the nervous system to reduce the movement of muscles in the stomach or intestine, and may be used for irritable bowels, as it also reduces muscle spasm. Possible side-effects: dry mouth, blurred vision, difficulty in passing water, rapid beating of the heart (palpitations).

Ranitidine *Zantac*

Reduces the production of stomach acid and may be used in the treatment of ulcers, reflux and some dyspepsias. You should not take antacids with ranitidine unless your doctor agrees. Possible side-effects: changed bowel habits, dizziness, rashes, tiredness.

Sucralfate *Antepsin*

This may be used in the treatment of ulcers or gastritis. If you have been advised to take antacids, you should not take them for at least half an hour before or after taking this medicine. Possible side-effects: constipation, diarrhoea, indigestion, dry mouth, rash, back pain, headache, dizziness, feeling drowsy.

Sulfasalazine [sulphasalazine] *Salazopyrin*

This may be used to treat ulcerative colitis or rheumatoid arthritis. Possible side-effects: feeling sick, headache, sore throat, fever, rashes, or you may pass orange-coloured urine (water). You should tell your doctor if you have fever, unexplained bleeding or bruising, a sore throat or if the medicine makes you feel weak.

Your Heart and Blood Vessels

Love may make the world go around, but it is the heart, arteries and veins that make the blood circulate. The heart is the main pump; the blood vessels are the tubes through which the blood runs to all parts of your body. Together they are called the cardiovascular system.

The heart has two halves, each with two chambers. The left half deals with blood containing oxygen, which goes by way of the arteries to the body cells. The right half receives the blood from the veins on its way back to pick up oxygen from the lungs. The system by which the blood goes between the heart and lungs is called the pulmonary system, or lesser circulation. (See also: Your Breathing System.)

The heart itself is made of special muscle tissue that can contract rhythmically without tiring. Its walls consist of a thick muscular tissue with membranes on either side. The heart walls contract, or pump, to the rhythm of a regular electrical message they receive from special tissue that acts as a pacemaker in the heart.

The blood flow in and out of the heart, and between its chambers, is controlled by valves that allow it to travel in one direction only. If the blood tries to flow back, it automatically closes the valve. The valves open and shut in time with the heart's pumping action to allow the blood to pass through.

Oxygen-rich blood is carried from the heart by a large blood vessel, the aorta. From it branch two coronary arteries that supply the heart muscle. Other branches, which themselves divide, supply the rest of your body with blood. The main arteries have elastic fibres that can expand and relax their walls. The arteries, through their smaller branches, carry blood to the capillaries, a complex network of micro-scopically small vessels through which the blood cells pass in single file.

The capillaries are threaded through all the tissues in your body. They supply the cells with nutrition from your blood. In their turn, the capillaries take waste matter from the cells and return it to your blood. The walls of the capillaries act as a barrier, keeping unwanted substances from passing from your blood to the cells, or vice versa. When the blood has given up its oxygen and nutrients, it flows from the capillaries into the veins for the return journey to the heart and lungs.

Also involved in this exchange system is a fluid called lymph. This fluid circulates through its own circuit (the lymphatic system) to the tissues. The lymph fluid exchanges nutrients for waste matter in the tissue cells. It also drains excess fluid from the tissues. The waste is filtered through the lymphatic system and eventually empties into the blood system for disposal.

Veins have thinner walls than arteries. They are also less muscular, and not as elastic. They contain valves which, like other valves in the circulatory system, ensure that your blood travels one way only. Venous (vein) blood is encouraged to flow by, among other things, the movement of your muscles that press against the veins, for example, in your legs and stomach. When you expand your chest to take in air during breathing, that also helps the blood in the veins to flow back to the heart.

While your blood is circulating round your body, it travels through several routes. At some time it has, for example, to filter through your kidney to be cleansed (the renal circulation). In your digestive system, blood picks up the food nutrients from the intestines. It flows through the liver (the portal system). The liver removes glucose (a sugar) to store and release when your body needs it. It also removes other substances that might be harmful to you. Other circuits through which the blood travels include the coronary circuit, through the arteries and veins of the heart itself. The circuit that sup-plies the neck, head and brain is called the cerebral circuit.

Everyone has blood pressure, whether it is normal, low or raised. The term refers to the force of the blood against the walls of the arteries. Several factors combine to cause blood to travel under pressure through your body. There is the force of your heart beat. It is also related to how elastic the walls of the blood vessels are and how easily they expand when blood is pushing through them. Hypertension is the medical term for persistently raised pressure; hypotension is low blood pressure. People with hypertension are more likely to suffer from strokes or heart attacks.

Common ailments

Diseases of the heart, arteries and veins are common among older people. However, by following your doctor's advice, many of the diseases can be controlled so that you can lead a normal, although slightly slower, life. The risks to people with diseases of the cardiovascular system are made greater by smoking and by drinking too much alcohol. You may also need to change your diet if you have heart, artery or vein problems. That will especially apply if you are overweight. Because the circulatory system is the transport system of your body, it is not surprising that, when it breaks down, other parts of your body are affected.

Varicose veins are swollen and knotted. They can be caused by long periods of standing or sitting, when there is not enough muscle action to encourage the blood to flow properly. The blood collects and presses back against the valves, causing the veins to swell. The valves no longer function efficiently, the blood collects and the veins gradually become more swollen and lose their elasticity. The result is a sluggish flow of blood. Women sometimes get varicose veins as a result of pregnancy. Phlebitis is inflammation of a vein.

'Arteriosclerosis' is a general word loosely used for a number of conditions affecting the arteries. In atherosclerosis, the artery walls are lined with fatty deposits, making a narrower blood channel. This can lead to parts of your body not getting the oxygen and nourishment they need. If the coronary arteries are affected, the supply of blood to your heart muscle will be reduced. If it happens in the cerebral arteries, the brain may not get enough oxygen and nourishment.

Ischaemic heart disease (shortage in the blood supply to the heart) is usually a result of narrowing of the arteries, and the same process is called peripheral vascular disease when it affects the limbs (usually the legs). The arteries also become stiffer and less elastic with age.

Blood clots sometimes form inside blood vessels, a condition called thrombosis. That can interfere with the blood flow. If a clot detaches itself from the walls of the blood vessel and is swept into the blood-stream, it is called an embolus. Fat globules and air bubbles also cause the sudden blocking of an artery, stopping the blood flow; this process is called embolism. If it affects the main artery between the heart and lungs, it is called pulmonary embolism.

Blockage of an artery in the brain is the main cause of a cerebro-vascular accident (stroke). A stroke may also be due to cerebral haemorrhage, bleeding from one of the brain's blood vessels. This may be linked to high blood pressure, to atherosclerosis or to a weak point on the blood vessel. With a stroke, parts of the brain may be damaged by a lack of oxygen-rich blood. It may then fail to send its electrical messages properly, causing problems with speech, memory or movements of the muscles, sensation of body, and control over bladder and bowels.

A transient ischaemic attack (TIA) is a temporary interruption of the blood flow to part of the brain. This may be due to an obstruction to the brain arteries, or to a spasm of the walls of the blood vessels.

Angina is the chest pain felt when the heart muscle is starved of oxygen-rich blood, because of narrowed coronary arteries. It often occurs when the heart beats faster with excitement or exertion, when the body uses up more of its 'fuel', oxygen.

Palpitations are when you can feel your heart beating abnormally rapidly. They can be a result of being over-excited or upset, or as a side-effect of some medications.

Cardiac arrhythmias are disturbances in the normal rate and rhythm of the heartbeat, which may cause palpitations. They happen when there is interference with the signals to the heart from its natural pacemaker. They can be due to chemical changes in the blood or some damage to the heart muscle, or may be an effect of some drug.

Tachycardia is the medical term for a heartbeat that has speeded up. Bradycardia is the term used when the beat has slowed down.

Congestive heart failure is when one or more of the heart's chambers do not empty properly. The blood then fails to circulate effectively.

A heart attack is a term popularly used to cover several types of serious heart problem. To doctors, a heart attack is a coronary thrombosis, which occurs when a blood clot blocks one of the coronary arteries. That stops the blood supply to an area of the heart muscle. It usually causes damage and permanent injury to the affected area.

Cardiac arrest is when the heart stops suddenly. It may be because the heart's pacemaker has stopped sending the electrical messages telling the heart to beat. It may also come after violent twitches (fibrillations) in the heart muscle. Immediate medical attention is needed when a heart attack occurs.

What medicines do

With problems of the circulatory system, you may need to take more than one type of medicine. Some treat the disease itself, while others treat the organs that the disease could damage. Some medicines may also be used to counteract the side-effects of prescribed drugs. In addition, some medicines may be prescribed to prevent new problems occurring. Several groups of drugs are used to treat diseases of the circulatory system. They include the following.

ACE inhibitors

This group of drugs may be used to treat raised blood pressure or heart failure. They act by interfering with the action of an enzyme that causes blood vessels to constrict (tighten). In this way, arteries are more able to widen, leading to blood pressure dropping. Possible side-effects: skin rashes, weakness, dizziness, loss of appetite.

Anti-arrhythmic drugs

These act to regulate the heartbeat and may be used when it becomes irregular or when it has speeded up (tachycardia).

Anticoagulants

These help to stop blood clots forming in your heart and blood vessels; they are also used to prevent and treat thrombosis.

Antihypertensive drugs

Such medicines reduce blood pressure. Diuretic drugs (see below) are also often used for this purpose.

Beta-blockers (beta-adrenoceptor blocking drugs)

These reduce the heart's work by blocking the action of adrenaline, a hormone produced during fear, anger or stress. They can be used for raised blood pressure, angina, arrhythmias and to prevent recurrence of a heart attack. Because they cause spasm of the breathing tubes, they are not suitable for people with asthma.

Calcium-channel blockers

These act on cells in the heart and blood vessels. They may help to reduce the force of the heartbeat or to relax the muscles in the blood vessels. They may be used for angina and raised blood pressure. It is thought that some calcium-channel blockers may be affected by grapefruit juice. If you are taking a calcium-channel blocker, it is therefore advisable to avoid drinking grapefruit juice. However, there is no evidence that eating the fruit (as opposed to drinking just the juice) causes interactions.

Cardiac glycosides

These are used to treat such problems as heart failure and a form of rapid heartbeat called atrial fibrillation. They slow down and regulate the heartbeat, blocking irregular useless signals, and the heart muscle action.

Diuretics

These act on the kidneys to remove water and salts from the bloodstream. In that way they increase the amount of urine passed, reduce the volume of blood and lower raised blood pressure. Various drugs of this type are listed in: Your Kidneys and 'Waterworks'.

Vasodilators

These relax and widen certain blood vessels, such as the smaller branches of the arteries, or they may be used to stretch the veins slightly. By doing that, it is easier for the heart to pump the blood. Vasodilators may be used in cases of heart failure.

Some other drugs and their brand names

Amlodipine *Istin*

This is a calcium-channel blocker (see also p 42) and may be used if you have angina or raised blood pressure. Possible side-effects: flushes, headache, ankle swelling.

Aspirin (low dose) *Angettes, Caprin, Disprin CV, aspirin dispersible tablets*, etc

This special low-dose aspirin may be used to help prevent blood clots forming in people with vascular problems or after heart surgery. You will not usually be prescribed this if you have a peptic ulcer, because you may risk a stomach bleed; check with your doctor. Possible side-effects: indigestion, which is less likely when aspirin is taken after food.

Atenolol *Antipressan, Tenormin*, etc

A beta-blocker (see also p 42), this may be used for raised blood pressure or angina. Possible side-effects: feeling sick, diarrhoea, tiredness,

Isosorbide dinitrate *Cedocard Retard, Isoket, Isordil, Soni-Slo, Sorbichew, Sorbitrate, etc*

A vasodilator, this may be used to treat angina or congestive heart failure. Possible side-effects: headache, flushing, dizziness, faster heartbeat.

Labetalol hydrochloride *Trandate*

This is a beta-blocker (see also p 42) that may be used for raised blood pressure and angina. Possible side-effects: tiredness, dizziness on standing up, sleep disturbances, headache, rashes, scalp tingling.

Lisinopril *Carace, Carace Plus, Zestril, Zestoretic*

This is an ACE inhibitor (see also p 41) that may be used to treat raised blood pressure or if you have had heart failure. Some brands contain a diuretic (see: Your Kidneys and 'Waterworks'), or you may be prescribed a diuretic medicine to take as well. Possible side-effects: rash, loss of taste, cough, sore throat, sore mouth, fever, dizziness, headache, tiredness, stomach upsets, mood changes, impotence.

Methyldopa *Aldomet, Dopamet, etc*

This is an antihypertensive drug (see also p 42). Possible side-effects: drowsiness, dry mouth, stuffy nose, depression. Men may have problems of ejaculation.

Metoprolol tartrate *Betaloc, Lopresor, etc*

A beta-blocker (see also p 42), this may be used for angina, raised blood pressure or arrhythmias. Possible side-effects: feeling sick, diarrhoea, tiredness, dizziness, sleep disturbances, cold hands and feet.

Nadolol *Corgard, etc*

A beta-blocker (see also p 42), this may be used to treat raised blood pressure, angina or arrhythmias. Possible side-effects: feeling sick, diarrhoea, tiredness, dizziness, sleep disturbances, cold hands and feet.

Naftidrofuryl oxalate *Praxilene*

A vasodilator, this may be used for problems affecting your circulation. Possible side-effect: stomach upset.

Nicardipine hydrochloride *Cardene*

A calcium-channel blocker (see also p 42), this may be used for angina or raised blood pressure. Possible side-effects: headache, flushing, dizziness, swollen hands or feet.

Nicotinic acid derivatives *Hexopal, Ronicol*

These are vasodilators. Possible side-effects: flushes, dizziness, feeling sick.

Nifedipine *Adalat, Adipine, Angiopine, Nifensar, Unipine, etc*

A calcium-channel blocker (see also p 42), this may be used if you have angina or raised blood pressure. Possible side-effects: headache, flushing, dizziness, swollen hands or feet, palpitations, feeling sick, increased need to pass water.

Oxprenolol hydrochloride *Slow-Trasicor, Trasicor, Trasidrex, etc*

A beta-blocker (see also p 42), this may be used for raised blood pressure, angina or arrhythmias. Possible side-effects: feeling sick, diarrhoea, tiredness, dizziness, sleep disturbances, cold hands and feet.

Pentoxifylline [oxpentifylline] *Trental*

A vasodilator, this may be used to treat circulation problems. Possible side-effects: feeling sick, dizziness, flushing.

Prazosin hydrochloride *Hypovase, etc*

This is an antihypertensive drug. Possible side-effects: dizziness, lack of energy, drowsiness.

Propranolol hydrochloride *Angilol, Apsolol, Bedranol, Berkolol, Inderal, Inderetic, etc*

A beta-blocker (see also p 42), this may be used for raised blood pressure, arrhythmias, angina or heart muscle damage. Possible side-effects: feeling sick, diarrhoea, tiredness, dizziness, sleep disturbances, cold hands and feet.

Verapamil *Cordilox, Securon, Univer*

A calcium-channel blocker (see also p 42), this may be used if you have angina or raised blood pressure. Possible side-effects: constipation, feeling sick, flushes, headache, dizziness, swollen ankles.

Warfarin sodium *Marevan, etc*

This prevents blood clots forming and may be used to treat thrombosis or embolism, or for people who have had heart valves replaced. Possible side-effects: it may cause bleeding of the gums, in the urine or as a nosebleed. If any of these happens, let your doctor or nurse know. With this medicine you should be given a treatment card by the doctor or pharmacist to remind you of the precautions.

Your Breathing System

Nearly all living creatures need oxygen to survive. All the cells in your body need it. The action by which you take in oxygen from the air and get rid of the waste gas, carbon dioxide, from the blood is called respiration – breathing in and breathing out. You need a change of air about 16–20 times a minute when you are awake, less when you are asleep and more if you have been taking heavy exercise.

Respiration begins when you take air in through the nose or mouth, where the air is warmed and moistened. Sinuses, cavities around the nose and eyes, may help in this process (although they also act as a sound chamber for your voice). In the nose, very small hair-like growths, called cilia, filter out dust and bacteria before the air goes through the pharynx (throat cavity), the larynx (voicebox) and down the trachea (windpipe). The windpipe has a sort of lid, the epiglottis, to prevent it taking in food when you swallow. (That should not be confused with the uvula, the fleshy part you can see hanging down at the back of your throat.)

The cilia (the small hairs) in the windpipe continually sweep foreign particles out of the breathing passages towards the mouth and nose. Particles too big for the cilia to deal with will be got rid of by a sneeze, the result of nerve endings in the nose being 'tickled', or by a cough when the nerve endings in the throat are stimulated.

From the windpipe, the air goes into the bronchi (air tubes). These branch out into the lungs where they further divide into bronchioles ending in millions of tiny air sacs or pockets (alveoli). The lungs are situated, along with the heart, in the chest cavity protected by the rib cage. The 'floor' of the rib cage is formed by the diaphragm, a thin muscle that divides the upper part of the body from the lower part containing the liver, stomach and bowels. The lung cavity is lined with a membrane, the pleura, which is a fine airtight skin that also covers both lungs. The space between the lining and the lung cavity is called the pleural cavity, although it is not a cavity in the conventional sense of the word; it provides just enough space for a film of fluid to allow the lungs to slide on the chest wall. The combined action of your ribs, their muscles and, importantly, your diaphragm helps you draw air into your body. As you relax, the air then leaves. Extra action to expel air, perhaps to blow out birthday candles, involves your chest and abdominal muscles.

The process of exchanging oxygen in the air for the carbon dioxide in your blood takes place in the tiny air sacs in the lungs. The walls of the air sacs allow the oxygen to pass through to the blood, which carries it round the body to the cells. In return, the blood gives up the waste gas, carbon dioxide, which passes through the walls of the air sacs in the opposite direction. The carbon dioxide then leaves the body through the mouth and nose, following the same route, in reverse, as the oxygen did as it entered your body.

Common ailments

Many older people suffer from respiratory problems, which are often most serious among those who smoke. There is no doubt that smoking causes some of the problems and, in all cases, makes them worse. If you have a respiratory problem, do not smoke. If you do smoke, try to stop: it is never too late to benefit from stopping smoking.

The respiratory system helps protect you by keeping out unwanted substances and germs in the air. When it breaks down, therefore, your resistance to germs is lowered and you may become prone to other illnesses. Problems of the respiratory system should not be taken lightly.

The common cold affects the upper part of the system. Membranes in the nose become affected and more mucus (fluid) than usual is produced. The inflammation can spread to your sinuses (sinusitis) and make your throat sore or cause a cough. Pharyngitis is inflammation of the throat cavity. Laryngitis is inflammation of the voicebox.

Infection spreading from the upper respiratory system can cause bronchitis, which is inflammation of one or more bronchi. But bronchitis can also be due to the irritating effects of substances that you have breathed in, such as dust, fumes or tobacco smoke. Bronchitis may be acute (sudden) or chronic (long-lasting). Inflamed bronchi will interfere with the amount of oxygen you take into your lungs. More mucus is also produced, and coughing to clear the mucus is needed to prevent it blocking your air passages, and also to prevent it gathering as a breeding-ground for more infection.

Emphysema is a lung disorder in which the small air sacs (alveoli) rupture or tear, join up, and become ballooned. They no longer function well, and the chest is kept inflated, so breathing – especially breathing out – becomes more difficult.

Asthma (sometimes called bronchial asthma) is also a condition in which breathing is difficult. The wheezing occurs because muscles in the bronchial walls constrict and narrow, especially when the person tries to breathe out. Asthma may be due to an allergy or it may come after repeated respiratory infections, or it may be a combination of the two.

Pneumonia is a disease that causes inflammation of a lung whose tissues become infected and blocked. Pleurisy, when the membranes surrounding the lungs become inflamed, makes breathing painful. It can be a complication of pneumonia. Several different bacteria or viruses can cause pneumonia, often as a complication of a cold or 'flu. It is also more likely in someone who spends long periods lying still on their back, when the base of the lungs becomes congested through not being expanded enough. Coughing, which is often painful, is needed to help your body get rid of the infected matter that gathers in the lungs.

Other diseases that affect the respiratory system include tuberculosis of the lung, and lung cancer. (See cancers in: Your Defence Systems, p 126.)

What medicines do

Medicines used to relieve coughs and the symptoms of cold and 'flu contain different drugs to reduce your discomfort. They may have only one or two ingredients, or they may contain several. If you intend to buy medicine for a respiratory problem, check with the pharmacist that it is suitable for you and will not interfere with other medicines you take. If you have been told to cut down your salt intake, you should also check that the medicine does not contain sodium. The same applies to sugar if you are a diabetic.

Cough suppressants (antitussives) are medicines that suppress a dry irritating cough that does not bring up phlegm (sputum). Expectorants are cough medicines that make sputum more watery and easier to cough up. Inhalants (medicines you breathe in) do the same. Decongestants unblock nasal, sinus or bronchial passages so that you can breathe more easily. Lozenges and linctuses help to soothe sore throats. (See also 'Vaccines' in: Your Defence Systems.)

Contained in remedies for coughs, colds, 'flu or catarrh, you may find some of the following drugs. You may want to ask the pharmacist which ones are suitable for your needs.

Analgesics

Aspirin and paracetamol are the painkillers most often included in this group. They are also used to bring down raised temperatures. Products containing aspirin should be avoided by people with peptic ulcers, stomach problems or asthma or who take medicines for blood disorders. Many cold and other remedies contain paracetamol, so you should take extra care that you do not accidentally take too much: an overdose of paracetamol can dangerously damage your liver.

Aspirin-containing medicines include: *Anadin, Beechams Powders, Phensic.*

Paracetamol-containing medicines include: *Beechams Powders Capsule Form, Benylin Day and Night cold treatment, Coldrex, Day Nurse, Lemsip, Medised, Night Nurse, Sinutab, Uniflu, Vicks Medinite.* Some products may contain both aspirin and paracetamol.

Antihistamines

These act on the nervous system to reduce the body's reaction in cases of allergy. If they cause drowsiness, do not drive a car or operate machinery. You should avoid products containing antihistamines if you are taking other medicines that act on the nervous system; check with the pharmacist if you are unsure. You should also avoid alcohol.

Diphenhydramine, promethazine and triprolidine are antihistamines that are often included in cough and cold remedies. Such medicines include: *Actifed products, Benylin products, Boots Cold Capsules, Boots Night Cold Comfort, Boots Night-Time Cough Relief, Dimotapp, Flurex Bedtime, Histalix, Night Nurse, Medised, Phensedyl Plus, Sudafed Plus, Tixylix Catarrh, Uniflu with Gregovite C.*

Bronchodilators

These act on the nervous system to open up the bronchial tubes. They are dispensed in a number of forms, including tablets and aerosol sprays.

Corticosteroids

These reduce inflammation and combat the effects of allergies. They may be dispensed in an aerosol spray or inhaler. They must be used regularly if they are to be most helpful.

Sympathomimetics

These act on the nervous system to relax bronchial muscles and allow easier breathing. They may have a stimulating effect on the heart and cause a rise in blood pressure. If you have raised blood pressure, heart disease, hyperthyroidism or diabetes, do not take such medicines unless your doctor prescribes them. They should not be used if you are taking, or have recently taken, drugs in the group called MAO inhibitors. (See: Your Nervous System.)

Phenylephrine, phenylpropanolamine and pseudoephedrine are the usual sympathomimetics found in the following list of cough and cold medicines: *Actifed, Beechams Powders Capsules with Decongestant, Benylin Cough and Congestion, Boots Decongestant Tablets, Catarrh Ex, Coldrex, Davenol, Dimotane products, Flurex Bedtime, Lemsip, Mu-cron, Sinutab, Sudafed products, Tixylix Cough and Cold, Uniflu with Gregovite C, Vicks Coldcare.*

Aerosol inhalers

Certain drugs prescribed for chest problems such as bronchitis, emphysema or asthma are often contained in aerosol sprays or inhalers. If you have been prescribed an inhaler, make sure that you understand how to use it so that the fine spray reaches down into your lungs. Your doctor or pharmacist will show you how to use it properly to get the full benefit of the medicine.

Sustained-release drugs

Some medicines, including some of those mentioned below, may be given as tablets or capsules known as sustained-release preparations. They act by releasing the medicine gradually into your system. Because they are specially prepared to work in this way, you should not crush or cut such tablets. For the same reason you should not chew them.

Unless you are instructed otherwise, take sustained-release medicines whole, with water, after food. Do not worry if the capsule's outer coating is passed in your stools; the medicine will have been absorbed by your body.

Some other drugs and their brand names

Aminophylline *Pecram, Phyllocontin Continus*

A bronchodilator, this may be used to treat asthma. Possible side-effects: faster heartbeat, feeling sick, stomach upsets, sleeplessness.

Astemizole *Hismanal, Pollon-Eze*

This antihistamine may be used to relieve the symptoms of allergies, such as hay fever. You should avoid this medicine if you have liver problems, if you already take anti-arrhythmic drugs, antipsychotic drugs, tricyclic antidepressants or diuretics. Alcohol is best avoided if you are taking this medicine. Possible side-effects: weight gain, skin rash, sleeplessness.

Beclometasone [beclomethasone] dipropionate *AeroBec, Becodisks, Becloforte, Becotide*

This is a corticosteroid that may be used in an inhaler for asthma. Possible side-effects: hoarse voice, mouth irritation.

Cetirizine *Zirtek*

This antihistamine may be used to relieve the symptoms of allergies, such as hay fever. Be cautious with alcohol, as it will have more effect on you when you are using this. Possible side-effects: tiredness, headache, drowsiness.

Ipratropium bromide *Atrovent*

This is a bronchodilator that may be used in an inhaler for chronic bronchitis. Possible side-effects: dry mouth, constipation.

Loratadine *Clarityn*

This antihistamine may be used to relieve the symptoms of allergies, such as hay fever. Alcohol is best avoided when you are using it. Possible side-effects: tiredness, headache, drowsiness.

Oxygen

In some cases of heart and lung diseases, oxygen may be prescribed by your doctor. In such cases, the oxygen should be thought of as a drug. It may be supplied in cylinders or be collected from the air in a piece of equipment called a concentrator. It is important to use it for the times and flow rates prescribed for you. Matches or naked flames should not be allowed anywhere near someone on oxygen therapy.

Salbutamol *Salbulin, Ventolin, Volmax, etc*

This is a sympathomimetic often used for bronchitis, emphysema or asthma. Possible side-effects: palpitations, hand tremors, nervous tension, headache.

Sodium cromoglicate [sodium cromoglycate] *Intal*

This is an anti-allergy drug that may be used to prevent asthma. Possible side-effects: cough, throat irritation.

Terbutaline sulphate *Bricanyl, Monovent*

This is a bronchodilator often used for bronchitis, emphysema or asthma. Possible side-effects: palpitations, hand tremor, nervous tension, headache.

Terfenadine *Aller-Eze Clear, Histafen, Seldane, Terfex, Triludan, etc*

This is an antihistamine that may be used to treat allergies such as hay fever, hives and skin allergies. You should not use it if you have heart problems or liver disease. You should avoid drinking grapefruit juice while you are taking this medicine. Possible side-effects: headache, indigestion, stomach pain. If you have heart palpitations or feel faint after taking terfenadine, you should see your doctor immediately.

Theophylline *Lasma, Nuelin, Slo-Phyllin, Theo-Dur, etc*

A bronchodilator, this may be used for bronchitis and emphysema. Possible side-effects: headache, faster heartbeat, feeling sick, stomach upsets, sleeplessness. Cough remedies that contain theophylline include: *Anestan, Do-Do Chesteze, Franol.*

Your Nervous System

Whether you are chewing an apple, walking, breathing or feeling happy, your nervous system is involved. Through various pathways to and from the brain, it is passing electrical signals to tell your tissues, muscles and organs what they should be doing.

The nervous system consists of the brain, the spinal cord and the nerves. They all act together as the communication and co-ordination system, carrying information to the brain and relaying instructions from it. By continually making adjustments and calculations, the nervous system keeps your whole body working in harmony.

The system has two main divisions. There is the central nervous system, which consists of the brain and spinal cord; and there is the peripheral nervous system, which itself is subdivided into the voluntary and autonomic systems. The autonomic system operates without your conscious control as the caretaker of the body. The voluntary nervous system controls the muscles and carries information to the brain.

The basic unit of the nervous system is the nerve cell, called a neuron. This highly specialised cell has many fibres leading from it. These fibres reach into muscles and organs throughout the body, to the ends of the fingers and toes. They cluster by the thousand in areas the size of a pinhead – for example, over your skin. The nerve fibres come together from the extremities of the body and gather in 'cables' running to and from the brain.

The spinal cord runs from about the top of the neck to the small of your back. Along the spinal cord are a number of 'relay stations' where nerves pass the signals from all parts of the body. These signals are sorted in the spinal cord and passed on to the brain to be analysed, acted on, linked with other information and sorted as memory.

The neurons that send signals to the brain from all parts of the body are called sensory neurons, contained in sensory nerves. Those that send signals from the brain to the muscles are called motor neurons, contained in motor nerves.

The largest part of the brain is called the cerebrum. That is divided into two halves, known as the right and left cerebral hemispheres. In turn, each hemisphere is divided into portions (lobes) with their own responsibilities.

Within the lobes are clusters of nerve cells that act as receiving centres. Each centre controls different parts of, or different functions within, your body. For example, one centre controls your heartbeat. Another controls your body temperature. A third controls your memory. And so on. Emotion, thought, mood and reasoning are all functions of centres in the brain.

Sensory centres interpret the signals from your senses of sight, hearing, smell, taste and touch. The sensory centres help you recognise such things as the difference between hot and cold, or sweet and sour. They tell you the shape and size of an object held in your hand. They sort out colours and sounds.

Information from the electrical signals can be transmitted between the brain's nerve centres. For example, the centre dealing with sight may link up with your memory centre. Thus if you see someone, the centres can communicate to let you know if you have seen that person before.

The different parts of the nervous system are continually in touch with each other. They are so well co-ordinated that you can think, feel and act on many different levels all at the same time. From the feeling of the outside air on your skin to the movements of your muscles, the flow of your blood or the mood you are in – the brain keeps track of everything affecting your body.

Two subdivisions of the autonomic system act to regulate the movements within your body so that they are not carried out to an extreme. These subdivisions work in harmony. One of them has generally a speeding-up effect. In response to danger or some other challenge, it almost instantly puts the body into a higher gear preparing it for any extra effort. The other subdivision acts to prevent the 'high gear' from being carried to extremes. It has a calming influence. Generally it acts as a damper, so that, unless the challenge demands a prolonged effort, the body processes will return to normal from their high gear. These systems of checks and balances are working all the time within your body.

All the electrical messages being transmitted to the brain happen at great speed. For example, if you place your hand on a hot surface, the nerves in your skin send a signal to your brain. Your brain signals back through nerves to the muscles. They then react to pull your hand off the hot surface. The stimulus of the hot surface leads to the whole series of reflex actions that cause you to remove your hand.

Other electrical signals are carried out without your conscious knowledge. These include such things as the signals that regulate your breathing, the operation of your digestive system and the secretions made by the various glands.

Each hemisphere of the brain sends and receives signals from the side of the head in which it is situated. However, the pathways of most motor nerves to your body cross over just about where your head and neck join. This means that the right hemisphere sends its signals to the left side of your body. Similarly, the left hemisphere sends signals to the right side of your body, including your right arm and leg. This explains why, after someone has had a severe stroke, the right side of the person's face is affected but it is the left side of the body that is afflicted, and vice versa.

Common ailments

Increasing age can bring with it a number of changes affecting the nervous system. The nerve cells may lose some of their efficiency and become slower at doing their job. During your lifetime they may have become damaged by accidents or disease.

As people grow older, there is often a slowing of the speed at which the electrical signals pass back and forth between the brain and the nerve endings in the muscles and tissues. That can lead to you taking longer to react – for example, to notice a pinprick on your finger.

You may also become less sensitive to changes in temperature so that you do not realise quickly that you are getting cold, or too hot. If you do not realise that you are getting cold, this can lead to a serious condition called hypothermia, which is when your body temperature falls below 35°C. Other causes of hypothermia include your body failing to regulate your temperature properly and your room or home not being warm enough.

The centres in your brain may be slower at sorting the messages they receive. Or they may misunderstand some of the signals. Your memory centres may take longer to record information or they may take longer to retrieve it.

Those parts of the nervous system dealing with sound, smell, taste or sight may become less efficient. So you may not hear as well as you used to, or be able to detect different smells as easily. Foods may also not be as tasty as when you were younger. Your eyesight may become a little poorer.

Some of these difficulties may arise because of a problem in the sensory pathways (those that send signals *to* your brain). Others may arise from problems in the motor pathways (those that pass signals *from* your brain) or in the connections between the two. They could also be a result of damage to the tissues, muscles or organs served by the nerve. Sometimes signals may be interrupted or altered by the effects of certain drugs needed to deal with other ailments you have.

Mental illnesses and other problems of the mind can have many causes. They may be organic (when brain tissues are injured or diseased). Or they can be caused by a lack of the body chemicals you need; or they may be due to too much of a chemical, such as alcohol, in your body. Alternatively, certain drugs may cause problems such as depression as a side-effect. Mind problems may also occur as a result of an ailment elsewhere in your body. The most common emotional illnesses are agitation, anxiety, confusion, depression, excitement, insomnia (sleeplessness), nervousness and tension.

Alzheimer's disease

Alzheimer's disease is one type of dementia (see below). It is a disorder of the mental processes, as a result of disease. It can affect your memory and your ability to reason. It may cause changes in your personality. Research is beginning to bring better understanding of Alzheimer's disease so that the symptoms may be controlled, even if the disease itself cannot yet be cured.

Dementia

Dementia is impairment of the thinking or understanding part of the brain. It may cause you to become confused. It can also involve disturbances of other functions, such as memory or the ability to perform certain tasks, and may lead to many types of unusual behaviour. Problems of speech are among the effects of such an ailment. Depending on their cause, some types of dementia can be treated and cured.

Epilepsy

Epilepsy occurs when the electrical messages in the brain become over-active. This is not a disease in itself, and the term is used to describe a group of symptoms that arise as a result of the sudden surge of electrical activity.

Neuritis

Neuritis, or inflammation of a nerve, has many forms. It may affect nerves in the peripheral nervous system – those that link the brain with the muscles, skin, organs and other parts of the body. With some types of neuritis, the part of the body served by the affected nerve may become more sensitive – a feeling of 'pins and needles' is an example. That can lead to pain. Other types of neuritis have the opposite effect, resulting in a loss of sensation or loss of function in an area of the body. Ophthalmic neuritis affects the nerve to the eye.

Neuralgia is a type of neuritis in which pain is the main symptom.

Trigeminal neuralgia affects a nerve in the head that has its nerve endings in the face and jaw. Sciatica is neuralgia in the sciatic nerve that runs from the spinal cord down the back of each leg.

Paralysis

Sometimes called 'palsy', paralysis is the loss of, or damage to, motor nerves, with the result that the cells in your muscles do not receive signals from your brain. Nerve diseases causing paralysis sometimes also cause disturbances of sensation. Depending on where the damage has occurred in the nerve pathway, a tiny or a large area of your body may be affected. Some types of paralysis are temporary, returning to normal when the disorder causing them has been corrected. Other types of paralysis may be more lasting.

Bell's palsy, which may last only a short time, is a paralysis of the facial nerve.

Hemiplegia is a paralysis affecting one side of the body, including the arm and leg. Paraplegia is a paralysis affecting both legs and possibly part of the trunk of the body.

Parkinson's disease

Parkinson's disease is due to a deficiency of dopamine in a small part of the brain. (Dopamine is a chemical compound produced in the body.) Parkinson's disease affects the nerve cells that transmit instructions to muscles in your body. It results in a breakdown in co-ordination between the brain and muscle cells, and can cause trembling, slurred speech or disturbance in any activity that calls for muscle co-ordination. It may occur without any known cause (called idiopathic Parkinsonism), or it may arise as a side-effect of some drugs.

Shingles (herpes zoster)

This is an infection of the ganglion, or relay station, of a nerve as it leaves the central nervous system. It is caused by infection with the chickenpox virus, which often lies dormant in the nervous system after an attack in childhood. The small blisters on the skin follow the path of the affected nerve or nerves.

Tic and tremor

Tic is an involuntary twitching movement of muscles that are usually under voluntary control. Tremor (trembling) may result from interrupted signals in the motor nerve pathways.

What medicines do

Many medicines have an effect on the nervous system, not only those that you take for problems directly affecting it. This is because with some ailments it is desirable to interrupt or, through chemical action, alter the brain's messages. For example, some analgesic drugs (pain relievers) act on the nervous system to reduce the pain messages to the brain from the part of your body that is hurt. Similarly, some medicines used to treat peptic ulcers may act on the nervous system to reduce the stomach's production of acids. (See also under the appropriate body system for other medicines.)

Analgesics

These pain-relieving drugs may be divided into three groups: those for mild to moderate pain; those for moderate to severe pain; and those for severe pain. Some analgesics also act to reduce inflammation.

ASPIRIN

Aspirin is an analgesic for mild to moderate pain. It should be avoided if you have peptic ulcers, stomach upsets or asthma, or are taking medicine for blood disorders. Possible side-effects: feeling sick, indigestion, rashes. Aspirin-containing analgesics include: *Anadin products, Aspro, Disprin products* etc.

PARACETAMOL-CONTAINING ANALGESICS

These are used for mild to moderate pain. Analgesics of this type include: *Boots Pain Relief Tablets, De Witt's Analgesic Pills, Hedex preparations, Panadeine, Panadol, Tramil,* etc. Many cough and cold remedies contain paracetamol, so you should take extra care that you do not accidentally take too much: even small overdoses of paracetamol can dangerously damage your liver.

IBUPROFEN-CONTAINING MEDICINES

These are used for moderate pain. You should not take these if you have ulcers or other stomach disorders. Possible side-effects: stomach upsets, water retention, tiredness, headache, dizziness. Analgesics of this type include: *Anadin, ibuprofen, Migrafen, Nurofen, PhorPain, Proflex, Relcofen,* etc.

MORPHINE-CONTAINING AND MORPHINE-RELATED MEDICINES

These analgesics may be used to control severe pain. Possible side-effects: feeling sick, constipation, drowsiness, lowered blood pressure, difficulty in passing water, dry mouth, faster heartbeat, hallucinations, mood changes. Analgesics of this type include: *diamorphine, MST Continus, Oramorph,* etc.

(See also analgesics in cough and cold medicines, in: Your Breathing System; and analgesics used for pains in joints, on p 93).

Types of mood-altering drug

Mood-altering drugs are sometimes called psychotropic or psychoactive drugs. Depending on their action they may be classed among one or more of the following groups.

ANTI-ANXIETY DRUGS

These are called anxiolytics, relaxants or tranquillisers, and act as sedatives (calming drugs) or as hypnotics (sleep-inducing drugs), depending on the dose. For that reason you may be prescribed an anti-anxiety drug as a sleeping tablet.

ANTIDEPRESSANTS

These act on the different symptoms whose underlying cause is depression. Such symptoms include low mood, anxiety, tension, appetite and sleep disturbances, loss of interest in life. The three main groups of antidepressant are those called SSRIs (serotonin selective re-uptake inhibitors), the group known as tricyclic antidepressants and the MAOI drugs (see below).

ANTIPSYCHOTICS

These neuroleptics or tranquillisers treat schizophrenia, paranoia and manic states. They may be used, in smaller doses, to treat agitation, anxiety or tension.

BARBITURATES

These calming and sleep-inducing drugs have largely been replaced by benzodiazepines, but phenobarbital [phenobarbitone] is still sometimes used in epilepsy.

BENZODIAZEPINES

These are anti-anxiety drugs, which may also be prescribed as sleeping tablets. They are habit-forming, and should, preferably, be taken for only a short period of time; when you stop, it should be under the supervision of your doctor. Possible side-effects: drowsiness, dizziness, unsteadiness, disturbances in muscle co-ordination, confusion, dry mouth, headache, vivid dreams, a 'hangover', skin rash. They may also affect your ability to drive or operate machinery.

MAOI DRUGS (MONOAMINE OXIDASE INHIBITORS)

These antidepressants block the action of monoamine oxidase, an enzyme that reduces the level of substances that control your mood. The drugs can have serious side-effects if taken with certain foods: a natural chemical in the food interacts with the drug and can lead to dangerously high blood pressure.

While you are on MAOI drugs, and for two weeks after stopping them, you must avoid cheese, liver and any offal, pickled herring and broad bean pods, for example. You must also avoid Bovril, Oxo, Marmite and similar foodstuffs, as well as alcoholic and even some low-alcohol drinks. It is advisable to avoid food that is stale or 'going off' – especially meat, fish, poultry, offal and game. You should be given a card to remind you of these precautions. Consult your doctor or pharmacist if you plan to take other medicines, including cold remedies and tonics, whether they are prescribed or bought over the counter.

SSRIs (SEROTONIN SELECTIVE RE-UPTAKE INHIBITORS)

This group of drugs increases the action of serotonin, one of the nervous system's chemical messengers. Medicines of this type may be used to treat depression. You should not take SSRIs if you are taking MAOI drugs (monoamine oxidase inhibitors) or if you have taken them within the past two weeks.

TRICYCLIC ANTIDEPRESSANTS

Normally, chemical messengers in the brain are constantly being released and then reabsorbed by brain cells. In depression, however, some types of chemical messenger may be produced in fewer amounts. Tricyclic antidepressants act to raise the levels of these chemical messengers by blocking the rate at which they are reabsorbed. Some tricyclic drugs act like a sedative, and so may be given if you have trouble sleeping. Others do not have this effect, and may be given to people whose depression makes them listless or lethargic. Possible side-effects: dry mouth, drowsiness, sweating, flushes, constipation, blurred vision, dizziness.

Some other drugs and their brand names

Amitriptyline hydrochloride *Domical, Elavil, Lentizol, Tryptizol,* etc

A tricyclic antidepressant, this is used to treat depression. Possible side-effects: dry mouth, bad breath, blurred sight, constipation, feeling sick, difficulty in passing water. It can affect your ability to drive or operate machinery.

Bromocriptine *Parlodel*

This is used for Parkinson's disease and also to treat gland problems. It should be taken at meal times, with your food. Possible side-effects: feeling sick, constipation, headache, dizziness (especially on standing up), drowsiness, confusion, disturbances in muscle control, dry mouth, leg cramps, stuffy nose, diarrhoea.

Carbamazepine *Tegretol*

This may be used for epilepsy, and also for trigeminal neuralgia and other painful nerve disorders. Possible side-effects: dizziness, drowsiness, stomach upsets, confusion, agitation, headache, impotence, double vision, rash.

Chlordiazepoxide *Librium, Tropium*, etc

A benzodiazepine, this may be given for anxiety. Possible side-effects: see 'Benzodiazepines' on page 65.

Chlorpromazine *Largactil*, etc

This is an antipsychotic drug used to treat schizophrenia. Possible side-effects: muscle tremor, hypothermia (lowered body temperature), drowsiness, dizziness on standing up, dry mouth, stuffy nose, faster heartbeat, rashes, nightmares, difficulty in passing water, impotence, blurred vision.

Clobazam *Frisium*

A benzodiazepine, this may be used for epilepsy or to treat anxiety. Possible side-effects: see 'Benzodiazepines' on page 65.

Diazepam *Tensium, Valium*, etc

This benzodiazepine is used to treat anxiety or insomnia. Possible side-effects: see 'Benzodiazepines' on page 65.

Domperidone *Motilium*

This may be used to treat nausea (feeling sick) and sickness if you have Parkinson's disease. Possible side-effects: muscle tremor, facial tics, skin rash.

Dothiepin *Dothapax, Prepadine, Prothiaden*, etc

This tricyclic antidepressant (see also p 66) may be used if you are ill with depression. Possible side-effects: dry mouth, bad breath, blurred sight, constipation, feeling sick, difficulty in passing water. It can affect your ability to drive or operate machinery.

Doxepin *Sinequan*

This is a tricyclic antidepressant (see also p 66). Possible side-effects: dry mouth, blurred sight, constipation, feeling sick, difficulty in passing water, sweating, speech problems, tremor, arrhythmias, faster heartbeat. In men, it may cause impotence.

Flurazepam *Dalmane*, etc

A benzodiazepine, this may be used to help you sleep. Side-effects: see 'Benzodiazepines' on page 65.

Haloperidol *Haldol, Serenace*, etc

An antipsychotic drug, this may also be given for severe anxiety. Possible side-effects: muscle tremor, hypothermia (lowered body temperature), dry mouth, stuffy nose, faster heartbeat, rashes. Men may have problems of ejaculation.

Levodopa-containing medicines *levodopa, Madopar, Sinemet*, etc

These are used to treat Parkinson's disease. Possible side-effects: confusion, loss of appetite, feeling sick, sleeplessness, agitation, dizziness on standing up, faster heartbeat, arrhythmias, drowsiness, depression, flushes, facial tics.

Lofepramine *Gamanil*

This is a tricyclic antidepressant that may be used if you have a depressive illness. Possible side-effects: dry mouth, bad breath, blurred sight, constipation, feeling sick, difficulty in passing water. It may affect your ability to drive or operate machinery.

Loprazolam *Dormonoct*

This is a benzodiazepine that may be used to help you sleep. Possible side-effects: see 'Benzodiazepines' on page 65.

Lorazepam *Ativan*

A benzodiazepine, this may be used for anxiety or sleeplessness. Possible side-effects: see 'Benzodiazepines' on page 65.

Lormetazepam

This is a benzodiazepine. It may be used to treat sleeplessness. Side-effects: see 'Benzodiazepines' on page 65.

Nitrazepam *Mogadon, Unisomnia,* etc

A benzodiazepine, this may be used to help you sleep. Side-effects: see 'Benzodiazepines' on page 65.

Orphenadrine hydrochloride *Biorphen, Disipal*

This treats problems of muscle control, including Parkinson's disease. Possible side-effects: dry mouth, thirst, stomach upsets, faster heart-beat, increased sense of well-being.

Oxazepam

A benzodiazepine, this may be used to treat anxiety and to help you to sleep. Side-effects: see 'Benzodiazepines' on page 65.

Paroxetine *Seroxat*

This SSRI (see also p 66) may be used if you have depression or get panic attacks. Possible side-effects: dry mouth, feeling sick, stomach upsets, diarrhoea, constipation, sweating, tremor, reduced appetite, rash, dizziness. It may cause sexual difficulties in men and women.

Phenobarbital [phenobarbitone]

Epilepsy may be treated with this. Possible side-effects: drowsiness, depression, rashes, excitement, restlessness, confusion.

Selegiline *Centrapryl, Eldepryl, Vivapryl,* etc

This may be used in the treatment of Parkinson's disease. Possible side-effects: sleeplessness, feeling sick, light-headedness, dizziness, vivid dreams, confusion.

Sertraline *Lustral*

This is an SSRI (see also p 66) that may be used if you have depression. Possible side-effects: dry mouth, indigestion, feeling sick, diarrhoea, tremor, drowsiness, sweating. It may cause sexual difficulties in men and women.

Temazepam

This benzodiazepine may be used if you have sleeping problems. Possible side-effects: see 'Benzodiazepines' on page 65.

Thioridazine *Melleril*

An antipsychotic drug, this may be used to calm you if you are restless or agitated. Possible side-effects: Parkinson's-like symptoms, hypothermia (lowered body temperature), drowsiness, sleeplessness, depression, disturbances in muscle control, hypotension (low blood pressure), dry mouth, stuffy nose, faster heartbeat, agitation, rashes, difficulty in passing water. Men may have problems of ejaculation.

Trihexyphenidyl hydrochloride [benzhexol hydrochloride]
benzhexol

This treats problems of muscle control, including Parkinson's disease. Possible side-effects: dry mouth, thirst, blurred sight, stomach upsets, flushes, faster heartbeat, constipation, difficulty in passing water. It may affect your ability to drive.

Zolpidem *Stilnoct*

Although it is not a benzodiazepine, this medicine acts in a similar way. It may be used to help you sleep. Possible side-effects: see 'Benzodiazepines' on page 65.

Zopiclone *Zimovane*

This acts in a way similar to the benzodiazepines, although it does not belong to that group of medicines. It may be used to help you sleep. Possible side-effects: dry mouth, bitter taste, stomach upsets, irritability, confusion, depression. (See also 'Benzodiazepines' on page 65.)

Your Glandular System

If you are crying with laughter, your tear glands are working; if you are perspiring with exercise, your sweat glands are at work. These glands, like most of those in your body, are called exocrine glands. They have ducts, or outlets, through which their secretions (fluids) are sent. In the case of the lachrymal (tear) glands, the fluids go to your eyes. With the sweat glands, the ducts open on to your skin. Other glands of this type include the sebaceous glands, which send an oily fluid to the roots of hairs. The prostate gland, a sex gland in men, is also an exocrine gland.

The other type of glands also at work in your body are the endocrine (or ductless) glands. These produce hormones, 'chemical messengers' that travel through your bloodstream to cells, tissues, muscles and organs. Hormones are an essential link in controlling your body's activities.

The chemical messengers are produced by the adrenal glands, the pituitary gland, the thyroid gland, the parathyroid glands, the thymus, the Islets of Langerhans in the pancreas, and the sex glands – the testes in men, or the ovaries in women. Some other body systems, such as the digestive system, also produce hormones, but these usually act only in the area of the body where they are produced.

Even though each of the endocrine glands has a specific job, they all depend on each other; and over-action or under-action by any one of them affects the whole endocrine system. The 'master gland' of the system is the pituitary gland.

Where the glands are

THYROID GLAND

Your thyroid gland is situated in the lower part of your neck, below your Adam's apple. Its hormones, which contain iodine, include one called thyroxine. This is sent into the bloodstream to help to regulate the speed at which the body cells use the energy fuel, oxygen. Thyroid hormones are important in regulating your body temperature.

PARATHYROID GLANDS

Your four parathyroid glands are situated near the thyroid. They produce parathormone, which acts to maintain the correct level of calcium and phosphates in your blood and bones. Teeth, as well bones, need calcium. It is also essential for the function of nerves, muscles and the heart.

ADRENAL GLANDS

Your two adrenal glands are situated near the top of each kidney. (That is why they are often called the suprarenal glands.) Each gland has two distinct parts, called the medulla and the cortex.

When you are excited, get a fright, or when the body has to make a special effort, a signal from the brain encourages the medulla to release adrenaline into your bloodstream. Adrenaline puts the body into higher gear for action. It increases your heart rate and speeds up the flow of blood. It widens certain blood vessels so that the oxygen in the blood reaches the muscle cells more quickly. It speeds up your breathing. It may cause more of the energy fuel, glucose, to go into your bloodstream, raising your blood-sugar level. Adrenaline also acts to widen the pupils of your eyes, so that they take in more light, and tightens your skin muscles, leading to 'goose pimples' and your hairs standing on end.

The medulla also produces a hormone called noradrenaline. That produces constriction (tightening) of blood vessels, leading to a rise in your blood pressure.

The cortex of the adrenal gland is directly controlled by a pituitary gland hormone. The cortex produces a large number of steroid hormones. Some steroids work directly with hormones from your pituitary gland to encourage your kidneys to retain sodium (a salt) and water. Others affect the rate at which your body uses up sugar. Steroid hormones, including one called cortisone, act to help your body deal with stress, such as injury or cold temperature. They also reduce the body's reaction to irritants or infections and can cause your body to retain salt and get rid of potassium. A number of the steroids are sex hormones.

ISLETS OF LANGERHANS

The Islets of Langerhans are specialised cells in the pancreas. They are concerned with producing insulin and glucagon, which work to control the level of sugar in your blood. When the level rises, the Islets send the insulin into your bloodstream to be carried round to the body cells. Insulin encourages the cells to take up some of the sugar from the blood, bringing the level back to normal. Because the sugar (glucose) is derived from carbohydrates, insulin plays an important part in processing the carbohydrates you eat.

Glucagon has the opposite effect to insulin. It influences the liver to release more glucose, raising your blood-sugar level. (See also: Your Digestive System.)

THYMUS

The thymus is an irregular-shaped organ that lies behind your breast-bone. It plays a part in your immune system that helps protect you from germs and disease.

PITUITARY

The pituitary is situated at the base of your brain. Its hormones influence the level of activity of nearly all the endocrine glands; for example, it stimulates the thyroid, and controls the adrenal cortex. The pituitary also influences the testes in men and the ovaries in women.

The pituitary's growth hormone is responsible for monitoring the size and number of the body's cells. It regulates developing bones, muscles and organs, and helps to determine your size and weight. It encourages your body to retain nitrogen. Growth hormone also affects the activities of your body cells. It can, for instance, influence the cells to slow down their intake of glucose, causing your blood-sugar level to rise.

Vasopressin is an anti-diuretic hormone produced by the pituitary. It encourages your kidneys to return water to the blood, instead of getting rid of it by way of the bladder. It is part of the sensitive system that controls the function of the kidneys and the level of water and salts in the body.

Also included among the pituitary gland hormones is oxytocin. That acts to squeeze muscles in the intestine and in the ureter, a tube linking the kidney and the bladder. (See also: Your Kidneys and 'Waterworks'.)

OVARY

The two ovaries are the sex glands of women. As well as producing eggs needed for reproduction, the ovaries produce hormones that influence women's sexual functions, such as menstruation (the regular monthly bleed), and feminine characteristics, such as breasts. The main hormones produced are oestrogen and progesterone. The natural production of oestrogen also protects women against both heart disease and a loss of bone density (osteoporosis). Progesterone helps prepare the endometrium (the lining of the womb) for pregnancy.

Between the ages of about 45 and 55 (although it can occur earlier and later), the ovaries stop producing eggs at regular intervals, reduce their production of oestrogen, and the monthly bleeds stop. This is known as the menopause. It may happen gradually over a period of years, when the time between bleeds gets longer, or it can happen quite suddenly.

PROSTATE

The prostate gland is an accessory sex gland in men. It lies just below the bladder. During ejaculation, it produces a fluid that forms part of the semen. (See also Your Kidney and 'Waterworks'.)

TESTIS

The two testes comprise the main sex gland in men. They produce spermatozoa (sperm), the male reproductive cells that are needed to fertilise a woman's eggs. Testosterone, essential for the development of male characteristics, is the main male hormone produced by the testes.

Common ailments

Diabetes or, to give it its correct name, diabetes mellitus, is probably one of the commonest problems affecting the glandular system. It is a condition in which there is a chronic (long-lasting) rise in the level of sugar in the blood. The Islets of Langerhans in the pancreas may not produce enough insulin, or the insulin being produced may not be as effective as it should be. In some cases, no insulin may be produced, perhaps as a result of disease or damage to the pancreas. Diabetes may also arise after an operation to remove part of the pancreas. In other cases, the body's defence system may be disturbed, leading it to attack the insulin it produces itself. Over a long period, diabetes affects other parts of the body. Eighty per cent of people with diabetes mellitus can control it by diet alone. Some of them, however, may need the help of sugar-lowering (hypoglycaemic) tablets. This type of diabetes is sometimes known as Type II or non-insulin-dependent diabetes mellitus (NIDDM). It is not fully understood why the condition arises, but it does tend to run in families. Other people may need to have daily doses of insulin, up to three times a day, injected under the skin. This type of diabetes is known as Type I or insulin-dependent diabetes mellitus (IDDM).

Deficiency means that there is none, or not enough, of a substance that your body needs. Thus, a hormone deficiency is a lack of a particular hormone. For instance, Addison's disease is an under-production of adrenal hormones. It may lead to a reduction of sodium chloride (salt) and water in the body, causing low blood pressure.

Cushing's syndrome is an over-production of the adrenal hormones. It can cause retention of water and sodium, and loss of nitrogen and potassium, and can lead to raised blood pressure.

Diabetes insipidus should not be confused with diabetes mellitus. Diabetes insipidus is a disorder that results from under-activity in part of the pituitary gland. Not enough vasopressin is produced, causing you to pass water frequently. As a result you are continually thirsty.

Ailments affecting the thyroid gland include goitre, which is an obvious swelling of the gland. Hyperthyroidism and thyrotoxicosis are related disorders associated with over-activity of the thyroid. Hyperthyroidism may cause 'staring eyes', loss of weight and shaky hands, but in older people, heart problems are more likely. Graves' disease is another condition associated with hyperthyroidism and goitre. Hypothyroidism or myxoedema is under-activity of the thyroid.

Problems affecting one of the parathyroid glands include hypoparathyroidism, a disorder caused by under-production of the parathyroid hormone. It causes a lowering of calcium in the blood. Over-activity of a parathyroid is called hyperparathyroidism. It may result in your body getting rid of too much calcium and phosphorus. It may cause kidney stones, sometimes caused by calcium collecting during the blood-filtering process.

For many women, the menopause is not a problem. For others, the change in the balance of the body's sex hormones can lead some uncomfortable symptoms. They include: hot flushes; your heart seeming to beat faster or louder; a dryness in the lining of the vagina, making sexual intercourse uncomfortable or painful; bladder irritation and infections; and various psychological difficulties.

What medicines do

To keep your endocrine system in order, medicines that affect one gland may need to be balanced by drugs that act on other parts of your body, including other glands. Different groups of drugs may be used to treat problems of the glandular system. Or they may be used to alter the chemical messages to the parts of your body where the problem occurs. In other cases, hormone drugs may be used to raise the level of hormones produced by under-active glands. That is often called 'replacement therapy'. Some sex hormones may be used in this way, either for men or for women. Drugs acting on your gland system include the following.

Corticosteroids

These are drugs similar to the hormones produced by the adrenal gland. Also known as steroids, they may be used to help replace hormones that your body is failing to produce. They may be used to act against allergies or asthma. Or they may be used to reduce pain and inflammation. (See also: Your Bones, Muscles and Joints.)

If you are taking steroid tablets, it is very important that they are not stopped, except under a doctor's supervision. This is because the adrenal cortex becomes less active during replacement. Depending on how long you have been taking steroids, it can take up to a year or longer to recover if a steroid drug is stopped; during that time the body is left with low hormone levels that could be fatal if not supervised.

You should always have a supply of steroid tablets in reserve. You will be given a card to carry with you at all times. If you consult a doctor, nurse, dentist or pharmacist, you must show them the card. Even after you have stopped taking the tablets, you must still inform them because the after-effects of steroids last a long time – up to several years.

If you have any other illness – a fever or diarrhoea, for example – you should see your doctor but do not stop taking the tablets. In fact, you may need an increased dosage at these times. You should also see your doctor immediately if the steroid tablets give you indigestion.

Possible side-effects: retention of water and sodium (salt); loss of calcium and potassium; raised blood pressure. Care must also be taken over accidents and infections, as steroids can reduce your body's ability to fight back.

Hormone replacement therapy (HRT)

In hormone replacement therapy for women, the female hormones oestrogen and progestogen may be used to relieve symptoms that can happen around the time of the menopause. HRT may be used if you have had an operation to remove your ovaries and/or womb. HRT to replace the protective hormone oestrogen may also be advised if you are at risk of developing osteoporosis, which affects the strength of your bones (see: Your Bones, Muscles and Joints).

For women who no longer have a uterus (womb), as a result of a hysterectomy operation, HRT using oestrogen alone may be acceptable. Those who still have a womb, however, face a risk of endometrial cancer (cancer of the lining of the womb) if they use oestrogen alone: for this reason, if you still have your womb you should use medicines that contain oestrogen and progestogen. This can be either two medicines or a single combined medicine containing both substances.

HRT to protect you against osteoporosis needs to be continued for a few years. Taken for a period of up to five years, the benefits of protecting you against osteoporosis, and possibly heart disease, seem likely to outweigh any risk of breast cancer. However, *after* five to eight years of using HRT, there is an increased risk of breast cancer. If you are aged over 60 and have used HRT for *more than* five years, the increased risk of breast cancer may be slightly greater. Because of that increased risk, if you decide to take HRT, you should preferably not be on it for any longer than five to eight years, unless you have discussed all the options with your doctor and agreed that it is right for you. Similarly, if you are at risk of thrombosis – if you have had thrombosis or if severe varicose vein problems run in your family, for example – using HRT may slightly increase that risk. In that case, you should decide with your doctor whether HRT is right for you.

Hypoglycaemic drugs

These are used to lower the level of sugar in your blood. When taken by mouth, they are called oral hypoglycaemics. Drugs of this type act in different ways: some stimulate your body to use up sugar, others are used to stimulate the release of insulin. Hypoglycaemic drugs must be taken at the specified times; if you miss or are late with a dose, check with your pharmacist or doctor.

Some other drugs and their brand names

Carbimazole *Neo-Mercazole*

This acts on the thyroid gland to treat hyperthyroidism. Possible side-effects: feeling sick, stomach upsets, skin rash, itching. You should tell your doctor as soon as possible if you experience pains in your joints, a sore throat or a raised temperature.

Glibenclamide *Daonil, Euglucon, Malix,* etc

This is an oral hypoglycaemic often prescribed for diabetes mellitus. Possible side-effects: feeling sick, stomach upsets, loss of appetite, putting on weight, too low a blood-sugar level (especially if taken late).

Gliclazide *Diamicron*

This is an oral hypoglycaemic used to treat diabetes mellitus. Possible side-effects: stomach upsets, loss of appetite, putting on weight, too low a blood-sugar level (especially if taken late).

Hydrocortisone *Hydrocortone*

A type of corticosteroid, this may be used in replacement therapy, perhaps needed as a result of Addison's disease. It also has a number of other uses (see p 113). **Important**: see 'Corticosteroids' on page 78.

Insulin

Diabetes mellitus is sometimes treated with this. It replaces the insulin the body cannot produce. The type of insulin, the dose and how often it is taken depend on individual needs.

Lypressin *Syntopressin*

This may be used as a nasal (nose) spray to treat diabetes insipidus. Possible side-effects: feeling sick, wind, stomach pains, urge to go to the toilet, stuffy nose.

Metformin *Glucophage, etc*

This is used to treat diabetes mellitus, in addition to dietary advice. Possible side-effects: loss of appetite, feeling sick, diarrhoea.

Oestrogen *Estraderm TTS, Evorel, Harmogen, Hormonin, Oestrogel, Ovestin, Premarin, Progynova, etc*

Medicines containing oestrogen may be used in hormone replacement therapy (HRT) for women who have had a hysterectomy. They may come as tablets, in a patch or as a gel. They should not be taken on their own if you still have your womb, as they increase the risk of cancer of the endometrium (the lining of the womb). If you still have a womb, oestrogen-containing medicine should be taken with progestogen-containing medicine. Possible side-effects: weight gain, feeling sick, sickness, breast tenderness; if you wear contact lenses, you may get eye irritation. (See also 'Hormone replacement therapy', p 78.)

Oestrogen and progestogen (cyclic) *Cyclo-Progynova, Estracombi, Estrapak 50, Femoston Patch, Menophase, Prempak-C, Trisequens, etc*

Medicines containing both oestrogen and progestogen may be used in hormone replacement therapy (HRT), especially for women who still have a uterus (womb). Regular bleeding, like periods, is likely to return. Possible side-effects: weight gain, feeling sick, breast tenderness, leg cramps. (See also 'Hormone replacement therapy', p 78.)

Oestrogen and progestogen (continuously combined) *Climesse, Kliofem, Premique, etc*

These may be used in hormone replacement therapy (HRT), especially for women who still have a uterus (womb). Because these are taken continuously, monthly bleeds (like periods) generally do not return with medicines of this type, although there may be some irregular bleeding when you first start taking them. Possible side-effects: weight gain, feeling sick, breast tenderness, leg cramps. (See also 'Hormone replacement therapy', p 78.)

Progestogen *Duphaston, Micronor, Provera,* etc

Medicines containing progestogen may be used in hormone replacement therapy (HRT) in conjunction with oestrogen-containing medicines, especially for women who still have a uterus (womb). Monthly bleeding (like periods) will return. Possible side-effects: weight gain, breast tenderness, blushing, depression, headache. (See also 'Hormone replacement therapy', p 78.)

Propylthiouracil

This acts on the thyroid gland to treat hyperthyroidism. Possible side-effects: feeling sick and stomach upsets, skin rash, itching. You should tell your doctor as soon as possible if you experience pains in your joints, a sore throat or a raised temperature.

Thyroxine sodium *Eltroxin*

This treats thyroid hormone deficiency. Possible side-effects: heart flutters, chest pain, faster heartbeat, muscle cramps, headache, restlessness, flushes, sweating, diarrhoea, loss of weight.

Tibolone *Livial*

This may be given to relieve some symptoms of the menopause. Possible side-effects: changes in your weight, spots, rash, itching, slight hair growth on your face, headache, dizziness, disturbed sight, ankle swelling.

Tolbutamide *Rastinon*

An oral hypoglycaemic drug, this may be used, in addition to dietary advice, to treat diabetes mellitus. Possible side-effects: dizziness, stomach upsets, loss of appetite, confusion.

Your Kidneys and 'Waterworks'

Your waterworks are only part of the urinary system, which could be called the body's main cleansing system even though your skin and breathing systems also get rid of waste matter in the body. The most important organs of the urinary system are your two kidneys. They filter the blood, getting rid of impurities, excess chemicals and waste matter in fluid form, as urine (your water). The kidneys also keep a proper balance between the electrolytes (salts) and the water in the blood. They help prevent the body fluids from becoming too acid. They manufacture hormones to help them in their task.

Your kidneys are situated just about waist level, close to the spine (backbone). Each kidney is linked by a tube, the ureter, to the bladder which is a storage bag that collects the urine. When the bladder is full, the urine passes through another, shorter tube, called the urethra, to the outside of the body – a process that is called urination (passing water, peeing).

The kidneys are most important because no other organ in the body can get rid of so many of the waste products of the blood. Luckily, one kidney is able to carry out the process.

Blood arrives at each kidney by way of the renal artery. It spreads through the kidney, through the artery's smaller branches, to the capillaries. These form a complicated network of tiny blood vessels, where the filtering takes place. This removes from the blood waste products such as urea and uric acid, and excess salts such as sodium, potassium and chloride. In addition, water and certain salts are taken back into the blood, depending on what the rest of your body needs.

The blood is returned to the general circulation by way of the capillaries and the renal vein. The remaining water and other waste materials stay behind as urine.

Urine moves through a series of ducts into a collecting funnel in each kidney, which sends the urine down the ureter to be collected in the bladder. As the bladder fills and pressure on its walls increases, you then get the signal, or urge, to pass water. The more fluid you drink, the more you have to pass as the kidneys receive the hormone signals to adjust the balance of water and other substances in the blood. (See also: Your Glandular System.)

Although you have no conscious control over urine travelling from the kidney to the bladder, most people have control over emptying their bladder, usually several times a day. Like walking, bladder control has to be learned in infancy.

Mostly for men

In men, the urethra extends to the end of the penis. As well as acting as an outlet for urine, the urethra is the exit path for semen at orgasm.

Situated below your bladder is the prostate gland, through which the urethra passes. (Women do not have a prostate gland.) The prostate continually produces a fluid that makes up the bulk of semen. It is ejaculated through the urethra during sexual activities. At other times, the excess prostate fluid flows into the urethra and is expelled in your urine.

Special types of tissue, called erectile tissue, are contained in the penis. They fill with blood after a signal from your nervous system. That stiffens the penis, so causing an erection.

Mostly for women

In women, the urethra ends in an opening just in front of your vagina. The vagina leads up to your uterus (womb), which lies just above and slightly behind your bladder. From your womb, two tubes – the fallopian tubes – lead up to each of your two ovaries.

Common ailments

Problems affecting the waterworks often distress or embarrass people, despite the fact that most of us have them at one time or another. However, as you grow older, you may find that slowed reaction times mean there is a shorter time lag between getting the urge to pass water and having to empty your bladder. Doctors call this 'urgency'. A decrease in the water-saving efficiency of your kidneys may also mean that you have to empty your bladder more often.

Urinary incontinence, a tendency to wet yourself, can occur for many reasons. Your bladder may let go when you are excited, get a fright or lose consciousness. It may also happen slightly when you cough or sneeze, and be only a mild temporary loss of control. Check with your doctor if you have a tendency to wet yourself, even mildly, as this can often be put right.

In men, an enlarged prostate pressing on your bladder may lead to an interrupted flow when you are trying to pass urine. Or it may cause you to go frequently to the toilet, both during the day and at night. (See also: Your Glandular System.)

'Stress incontinence' occurs when a person coughs, sneezes, picks up something heavy or braces their tummy muscles for any reason. A small amount of urine then leaks out. In women it may result from gynaecological problems such as prolapse of the womb. That happens when slack muscles allow the floor of the womb to drop down into the vagina. A slackening of muscles at the outlet between the bladder and urethra is another cause of incontinence.

Waste matter (stools, motions, faeces) stuck in your bowel can cause pressure on your bladder, leading to urinary incontinence. Stools may then overflow; this is faecal incontinence. (See also: Your Digestive System.)

You can have problems with your waterworks as a result of damage along any part of the nervous system operating between your brain and your bladder – for example, after a stroke. A misdirection of some nerve signals may make you unsure whether you are emptying your bladder or your bowel, which may be particularly dismaying if you are a man.

Urinary infection may cause bladder irritation, giving you the urge to pass urine even when your bladder is empty. Some infections may cause pain when or after you pass water. Cystitis, often due to infection, is inflammation of the bladder. This can spread to your kidneys and ureter. (See also: Your Defence Systems.)

Both urinary frequency and incontinence can also be a side-effect of medicines.

Some problems with your kidneys can be caused by kidney stones. These are usually due to calcium forming around a blood clot, fat globule or bacteria. A few are due to an excess of calcium in your blood. Nephritis is inflammation of a kidney.

An upset in your glandular system can lead to your kidneys getting the wrong message from hormones, causing an imbalance of salts or other substances in your blood. Nephrosis is a condition in which kidneys lose their control over the water content of the blood. That can lead to water being retained in your body cells and tissues, a condition called oedema. Uraemia is a condition caused by kidney failure when urea, a waste product, does not get expelled by your kidneys. As a result, urea and other waste matter build up in your blood.

Tumours may also occur in the urinary system. They can often be treated and kept under control for many years.

What medicines do

Among the medicines affecting the urinary system, probably those used most frequently by older people are the drugs known as diuretics (water tablets). Diuretics act to encourage your kidneys to get rid of water and salts from your blood. They may be used to lower your blood pressure by reducing the amount of salt in the body. They may be used to treat heart failure by reducing the volume of blood, and thus the amount of work that the heart has to do. Diuretics are also prescribed for oedema, perhaps because of liver or kidney ailments.

Some diuretics act to reduce the amount of sodium the kidneys return to your bloodstream. They may also reduce the amount of potassium it contains. For that reason, you may have to be given potassium supplements to bring the level back to normal (see p 119 in: Your Blood and Nutrition). Many diuretics are combined in tablets with other medicines. Diuretics are usually taken in the morning so that the need to empty the bladder doesn't disturb sleep.

Thiazide diuretics

This is the name given to a group of diuretic drugs that may be used to treat water retention or raised blood pressure (hypertension). Some thiazide diuretics may cause you to lose potassium, in which case you may be given a potassium supplement as well. Possible side-effects: rashes, stomach upsets, dizziness, loss of appetite. Gout and diabetes or, in men, impotence are also possible side-effects.

Some other drugs and their brand names

Amiloride hydrochloride *Amilospare, Berkamil,* etc

A diuretic drug, this may be used to treat water retention or to help retain potassium. Possible side-effects: rashes, thirst, feeling sick, dizziness, confusion.

Bendroflumethiazide [bendrofluazide] *Aprinox, Berkozide, Neo-NaClex,* etc

This is a thiazide diuretic that may be used to treat water retention or high blood pressure. Possible side-effects: see 'Thiazide diuretics', above.

Bumetanide *Burinex*

A diuretic drug, this may be used to treat water retention. Possible side-effects: dizziness, feeling sick, stomach upsets, rashes, joint pains.

Clortalidone [chlorthalidone] *Hygroton*

A diuretic drug that is similar to thiazides (see above), this may be used if you have water retention, high blood pressure or diabetes insipidus. Possible side-effects: rashes, thirst, stomach upsets, headache, dizziness; impotence in men.

Cyclopenthiazide *Navidrex*

This is a thiazide diuretic that may be used to treat water retention or high blood pressure. Possible side-effects: see 'Thiazide diuretics' on page 87.

Distigmine bromide *Ubretid*

This acts on your nervous system to relieve urinary retention. It may be used if you have bladder problems due to nerve damage. Possible side-effects: feeling sick, sickness, sweating, blurred sight, mouth-watering, slower heartbeat, wind, diarrhoea.

Finasteride *Proscar*

This acts on the prostate gland and may be used to relieve symptoms if you have an enlarged prostate. It is important that crushed or broken finasteride tablets should not be handled by women who are (or who may become) pregnant, because contact with finasteride can cause abnormalities in unborn males. If you are taking finasteride and have a partner who could become pregnant, you should also wear a condom as your semen will contain traces of the drug. Possible side-effects: reduced sex drive, impotence, lip swelling, skin rash.

Flavoxate hydrochloride *Urispas*

This acts on your bladder muscle to treat problems of incontinence. You should avoid it if you have glaucoma. Possible side-effects: headache, feeling sick, tiredness, blurred sight, dry mouth, diarrhoea.

Furosemide [frusemide] *Dryptal, Froop,* etc

A strong diuretic drug, this may be used for water retention. You may also be given a potassium supplement with this medicine. Possible side-effects: dizziness, rashes, ringing in your ears, cramps.

Hydrochlorothiazide *Dyazide, HydroSaluric, Moduretic*

This is a thiazide diuretic that may be used to treat water retention or high blood pressure. Possible side-effects: see 'Thiazide diuretics' on page 87.

Lubricating jelly *KY Jelly, etc*

This is a sterile (germ-free) gel that may be used as lubrication for women, to prevent painful sexual intercourse. Doctors and nurses also use it to help with internal examinations.

Spironolactone *Aldactone, Laractone, Spirolone, Spirospare, etc*

This is a diuretic drug that may be used if you have fluid retention, a kidney or liver problem, or heart disease. It may be given as well as other diuretic medicines. Possible side-effects: feeling sick, headache, sleepiness, rash, impotence.

Terazosin hydrochloride *Hytrin BPH*

This acts to relax the muscle of the prostate gland and bladder. It belongs to the group of drugs known as alpha-blockers. It may be used for raised blood pressure. If you are allergic to alpha-blockers you should not take this medicine. Possible side-effects: headache, dizziness, weakness, feeling sick, faster heartbeat, weight gain, drowsiness, blocked nose, blurred vision, impotence. It may affect your ability to drive.

Triamterene *Dytac, Dytide, Frusene, Kalspare, etc*

A diuretic drug, this may be used if you have raised blood pressure or water retention or if you need to retain more potassium. Possible side-effects: stomach upsets, dry mouth, rashes. It may turn your urine (water) slightly blue.

Your Bones, Muscles and Joints

Whatever basic shape you are – tall or short, broad or narrow – you owe to your bones. They are the framework of your body. Their joints allow you to move. Your muscles provide the means of moving. Together they are called your musculo-skeletal system.

Your bones give your body support and strength, as well as shape. They also act as a store for the calcium the rest of your body needs.

In hollows in some bones, such as parts of your skull, your ribs and the bones in your spine, is a substance called marrow. Marrow is a spongy material containing a network of blood vessels and special tissues. They hold together fat and cells that manufacture blood cells.

The bones in your body meet at joints. Some joints do not move, such as those in your skull that have fused together to protect the brain. Where there is movement, the joints are of different types to allow your body to move in various ways. A fine skin-like material (membrane) lines and protects the ends of bones where they meet. Called the synovial membrane, it lubricates the joint with synovial fluid. The surfaces of the mobile joints are covered by a special type of tissue, called cartilage.

In your vertebral column (spine, backbone) the rings of cartilage between the vertebrae (bones) are known as discs. Inside the vertebral column, and protected by the bones, is your spinal cord.

Bones are moved at their joints by your muscles. These are bundles of long thin cells (fibres) that can tense and relax to produce movement. Some muscles are attached directly to your bones. Others are attached by extra-strong fibres (tendons). Muscles may be attached to each other. Or they may link your skin and bones, as in some muscles in your face. Muscles can be very strong, like those of your thighs, or your back muscles, which give you posture. Or they can provide delicate movements, such as those that turn your eyes.

Each muscle fibre receives its own signals through your nervous system. Each has its own store of energy food, glycogen, which, together with oxygen and other nutrients, is brought to it by the blood. The muscle fibre's waste products are passed into the bloodstream for disposal.

Although you have muscles in other parts of your body, such as your intestine and heart, those that are concerned with movements of your bones and joints are called skeletal muscles. They are under your deliberate control, through your voluntary nervous system. Groups of muscle act as a team to perform the movements you make, whether it is walking, chewing or playing the piano.

Common ailments

Age does not necessarily bring with it aches and pains in muscles and bones, but certain ailments are found more among older people than the young. Pain is an indication that something is wrong and should be checked with your doctor. Arthritis and rheumatism are the names most people give to the pains and stiffness affecting their muscles, bones and joints. Strictly speaking, however, that is not quite correct. Arthritis is inflammation of a joint. Rheumatism covers a variety of diseases involving inflammation and changes in the structure of muscles, bones, cartilage or joint membranes. The two main types of joint ailment are osteoarthritis and rheumatoid arthritis.

Osteoarthritis involves a breakdown of cartilage that covers a joint. As the cartilage wears away, the surface of the bones becomes less protected. Part of the bone may wear away and there may be changes in the synovial membrane. Osteoarthritis is most likely to affect the joints that have received most use over the years – your hips or knees, for example.

Rheumatoid arthritis is an ailment affecting many of the connective tissues throughout your body. Joints may become red and swollen. It can also affect the synovial membrane and destroy the cartilage. Bones may be damaged, and their cell-making ability can be affected. As well as changes in the joints and bones, the muscles and skin near them are all likely to be affected. Both problems can be painful and lead to the affected area becoming misshapen. Other parts of the body, such as the lungs, can also be affected.

Gout is also a type of arthritis. With it, an excess of uric acid in the blood leads to urate micro-crystals being deposited in joints and tissues.

Ailments mainly affecting bones include fractures (breaks) and osteoporosis. Osteoporosis is a thinning of the bones, which become less strong than before, and liable to break more easily. A minor fall can lead to a fracture, most commonly of the hip, spine or wrist. It affects both men and women, but is more common and more severe in women because of a lack of the female hormone oestrogen after the menopause. Among men, it is sometimes due to low levels of the male hormone testosterone. Not enough calcium in your diet may make things worse. It can be linked to other diseases, and it may be a side-effect of long-term use of some drugs, such as corticosteroids, or excess alcohol consumption, or tobacco smoking. Some doctors think it may be made worse by consuming too much salt in food, including processed foods. Bones in older people may not repair themselves as quickly as young bones. (See also: Your Glandular System.)

A type of rickets in adults, called osteomalacia, may be due to a lack of vitamin D, reducing your body's absorption of calcium. As a result, your bones may become less firm. Vitamin D is found in foods such as fish, cod liver oil, margarine and liver but it is mainly made in the skin on exposure to sunlight. Osteomalacia is therefore more common in house-bound older people with a poor diet. Some medicines can affect how your body absorbs vitamins and minerals. (See also: Your Blood and Nutrition.)

Paget's disease is a condition affecting your bones. It can lead to some bones becoming thickened and deformed, and may cause pain. It may affect the bones of your skull, your backbone (spine), hips (pelvis) and the long bones in your arms or legs.

As you grow older, your skeletal muscles tire more easily and you may not be as agile as you were. Your muscles may also become smaller, partly because they are not used as much. Tendons may also shrink.

Muscle cramps and 'pins and needles' are common complaints and can happen at any age. Fibrositis is inflammation in a muscle.

What medicines do

Many of the medicines used to treat ailments affecting your muscles, bones and joints aim to reduce pain and inflammation and stiffness. Other medicines may be used to help prevent ailments affecting your bones, such as HRT for osteoporosis (see 'Hormone replacement therapy' on p 78 in: Your Glandular System). Some medicines may be given as suppositories, which are inserted into the rectum (pushed gently up your bottom). If you are given these, ask your doctor, nurse or pharmacist how to use them.

Analgesics are pain-relieving drugs. Anti-inflammatory drugs reduce swelling. Rubefacients, medicines that you rub into your skin, may be used to relieve stiffness and ease pain. (See also: Your Skin.)

Aspirin, paracetamol, codeine and ibuprofen are four drugs contained in a number of medicines you may buy to relieve muscle aches and pains. Products containing aspirin, and most NSAIDs (see p 94), should be avoided by people with peptic ulcers or stomach problems, or those who take medicines for blood disorders. Many people, particularly those with a history of asthma, are allergic to aspirin. Products containing paracetamol have no effect on inflammation and stiffness. Products containing codeine phosphate can lead to constipation.

Aspirin-containing medicines

These include: *Aspro, Caprin, Disprin, Fynnon Calcium Aspirin, Phensic*, etc. Medicines containing aspirin should be avoided if you have peptic ulcers, stomach upsets or asthma, or are taking medicines for blood disorders.

PARACETAMOL-CONTAINING MEDICINES

These include: *Co-dydramol, Hedex, Panadol*, etc. Many cough and cold remedies contain paracetamol, so you should take extra care that you do not accidentally take too much. Even small overdoses of paracetamol can dangerously damage your liver.

ASPIRIN AND CODEINE PHOSPHATE-CONTAINING MEDICINES

These include: *Co-codaprin, Codis*, etc. Medicines containing aspirin should be avoided if you have peptic ulcers, stomach upsets or asthma, or are taking medicines for blood disorders.

PARACETAMOL AND CODEINE PHOSPHATE-CONTAINING MEDICINES

These include: *Co-codamol, Panadeine, Paracodol, Syndol*, etc. Many cough and cold remedies contain paracetamol, so you should take extra care that you do not accidentally take too much. Even small overdoses of paracetamol can dangerously damage your liver.

IBUPROFEN-CONTAINING MEDICINES

These include: *Advil, Novaprin, Nurofen, PhorPain*, etc. See also 'NSAIDs', below.

NSAIDs (non-steroidal anti-inflammatory drugs)

This group of drugs may be used to reduce pain and swelling in your joints, perhaps if you have rheumatoid arthritis or osteoarthritis, or for an acute attack of gout. They are given their name to distinguish them from the group known as corticosteroids (see 'Corticosteroids' on p 78 in: Your Glandular System). NSAIDs can irritate the stomach, and should be taken after food. They are not suitable for people with peptic ulcer. Aspirin and ibuprofen are NSAIDs that may be contained in remedies you can buy over the counter. You should not take more than one medicine that contains an NSAID unless you have first discussed this with your doctor.

Bisphosphonates

Bisphosphonates are a group of drugs that may be used to treat Paget's disease, or in the treatment of osteoporosis in women who have passed the menopause. They act to slow down bone loss.

Some other drugs and their brand names

Alendronic acid *Fosamax*

This is a bisphosphonate that may be used to treat osteoporosis. If you get pain after swallowing this medicine, or heartburn after taking it, you should tell your doctor as soon as possible. You should take this medicine with a full glass of water and not lie down for at least 30 minutes after taking it. You should not take it at bedtime. Possible side-effects: stomach pain, diarrhoea, constipation, wind, aches, headache, rash.

Allopurinol *Caplenal, Cosuric, Xanthomax, Zyloric,* etc

This may be used to prevent gout. You should drink plenty of fluid if you are prescribed this medicine. Possible side-effects: rashes, stomach upsets, sleepiness, headache, vertigo.

Auranofin *Ridaura*

This may be used if you have rheumatoid arthritis. Possible side-effects: diarrhoea, feeling sick, stomach pains, sore throat, mouth ulcers, rash, bruising, high temperature. You should see your doctor immediately if you get any of these.

Benorylate *Benoral*

This is derived from aspirin and paracetamol (see pp 93 and 94).

Co-proxamol *Cosalgesic, Distalgesic*

Pain and inflammation may be treated with this. It contains paracetamol. Possible side-effects: stomach upsets, feeling sick, constipation, sleepiness, confusion, unsteadiness and falls.

Diclofenac sodium *Rhumalgan, Voltarol*, etc

This NSAID may be used to reduce pain and inflammation. Possible side-effects: stomach upsets with pain and diarrhoea, rashes, water retention, tiredness, dizziness, headache.

Disodium etidronate *Didronel PMO*

This bisphosphonate may be used in Paget's disease or to treat osteoporosis. For two hours before and after taking this medicine, you should not take any foods, particularly calcium-containing foods or milk. You should also avoid antacids, and iron and mineral supplements. You should not take this medicine for more than three years unless you have discussed this with your doctor. Possible side-effects: feeling sick, diarrhoea, itching, headache, stomach ache, constipation.

Fenbufen *Lederfen*

This NSAID is used to treat pain and inflammation in rheumatic diseases. Possible side-effects: stomach upsets, loss of appetite, heartburn, diarrhoea, constipation, tiredness, dizziness, headache, swelling of your face or feet, sight disturbances. If you get a rash or are short of breath, you should stop taking this medicine and see your doctor as soon as possible.

Fenoprofen calcium *Fenopron, Progesic*

This is an NSAID used to reduce pain and inflammation. Possible side-effects: stomach upsets, diarrhoea, constipation, mouth ulcers, dry mouth, metallic taste, rashes, water retention, tiredness, dizziness, headache.

Flurbiprofen *Froben*

This NSAID may be used to reduce pain and inflammation and to treat gout. Possible side-effects: stomach upsets, rashes, water retention, headache, tiredness, dizziness.

Ibuprofen *Apsifen, Brufen, Fenbid, Lidifen*, etc

This is an NSAID that may be used to reduce pain and inflammation.

Possible side-effects: stomach upsets, water retention, tiredness, dizziness, rashes, headache.

Indometacin [indomethacin] *Artracin, Imbrilon, Indocid,* etc

Pain and inflammation may be treated with this NSAID, which may also be used to treat gout. Possible side-effects: headache, dizziness, light-headedness, stomach upsets, confusion, blurred sight, depression, tiredness, sleeplessness, ringing in your ears. It can affect your ability to drive or operate machinery.

Ketoprofen *Orudis, Oruvail*

This NSAID may be used to reduce pain and inflammation. Possible side-effects: stomach upsets, rashes, water retention, tiredness, dizziness.

Naproxen *Arthroxen, Naprosyn, Nycopren,* etc

Used to reduce pain and inflammation, this NSAID may also be used to treat gout. Possible side-effects: stomach upsets, rashes, water retention, tiredness, headache, dizziness.

Piroxicam *Feldene, Larapam,* etc

This is an NSAID that is given in the treatment of pain and inflammation or for gout. Possible side-effects: stomach upsets, water retention, dizziness, headache, rashes, tiredness.

Prednisolone *Deltacortil, Precortisyl, Prednesol,* etc

This is a corticosteroid that acts on many parts of the body, including the glandular system. It may be used to reduce joint inflammation. Possible side-effects: osteoporosis, diabetes, depression. **Important**: see 'Corticosteroids' on page 78 in: Your Glandular System.

Quinine sulphate

This may be used to relieve night cramps in the legs. Possible side-effects: tinnitus (ear noise), headache, stomach upsets, feeling sick, sight disturbance, confusion.

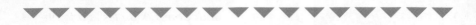

Your Special Senses

Collecting information from the world outside your body is the job of your senses of sight, hearing, smell, taste and touch. They all send signals to your brain so that you are aware of what is going on around you. Sight, hearing, smell and taste are covered in this chapter; touch is mentioned in the next chapter: Your Skin.

SIGHT

Your visual system, which enables you to see, has three main parts. They are: your eye; the visual centre in your brain; and the optic nerve which connects the two.

Your eyeball has three 'coats'. The outer layer of tough tissue gives it shape and protects the delicate inner layers. The eye muscles that allow you to move your eyes are attached to the outer layer. The middle 'coat' contains the main arteries and veins of the eyeball. The inner 'coat' is the retina, containing many nerve cells.

The eyelids protect your eye. They are lined by a protective membrane called the conjunctiva, which also covers and protects the surface of your eyeball. Lachrymal glands make tears to wash and lubricate the surface of your eye. The tears drain away through ducts. If there are too many tears to drain away, they do, of course, flow over the lower lid, as, for example, when you cry.

Your eye works as a camera does, and it needs light to function. The light first passes through a transparent window called the cornea before it reaches the iris, a muscle whose colour determines whether you have blue, brown, green or grey eyes. In the centre of the iris is a hole called the pupil. As in a camera, the pupil can be narrowed or widened (dilated) to control the amount of light going through. Behind the iris is the lens that directs and focuses the light on to a screen, the retina, that lines the back of the eye. The retina reacts to the light and changes it into electrical messages. These are sent through the optic nerve to the visual centre in your brain. That interprets the messages and conveys them to other brain centres.

The space between the lens and the cornea contains aqueous humour, a watery fluid that maintains an even pressure inside the eyeball to help it keep its shape.

The retina perceives, through the messages of light, the colour of an object. To bring an object into focus on the retina, whether the object is near or distant, involves adjustments of the lens by the muscles attached to it.

Common ailments

Eyesight changes as you grow older, as most people become aware when they find they have to use reading glasses for the first time. Over the years, the lens gradually loses some of its elasticity and changes its shape. It then becomes too rigid to focus print at the normal reading distance. The cornea, too, may alter slightly. The white outer layer also grows slightly harder. And less of the watery fluid, aqueous humour, is produced. These changes in the eye alter the way it focuses, which is why it is sensible to have a sight test once a year.

Your eyes may no longer be able to accommodate such a wide range of light conditions – from the very bright to the very dim. That may lead to some lights seeming too strong. Others may not be strong enough or more light may be needed when reading or doing close, delicate work. Some colours may not be so easily distinguished.

Tear glands may produce fewer tears, leading to dry eyes. Eyelid tissue may become thinner. Watery eyes may be due to a blockage of the tear duct, or sagging of the lower lid.

Some eye problems are caused by other ailments. For example, raised blood pressure may cause bleeding in tiny blood vessels in the eyes.

Problems or disturbances affecting parts of your nervous system can also have an effect on the signals between your brain centre and your eye. Some drugs may have side-effects on the eyes. For example, there are drugs used for digestive ailments and urinary problems that can enlarge the pupil, so that the squashed-up iris prevents the aqueous fluid draining away. That raises pressure inside the eyeball, a condition called glaucoma.

A cataract is opacity of the lens – that is, it becomes less transparent.

Conjunctivitis is inflammation of the conjunctiva, perhaps through infection or injury.

A detached retina is exactly what it suggests, part of the retina has come loose from its base.

Eyestrain is tiredness of the eye. That may be due to improper use, such as reading too long in a poor light. Or it may be an effect of eye ailments.

Macular degeneration is a disease that destroys part of the retina of the eye. As a result, the central part of your sight is impaired, although vision at the edges may be less affected.

Retinopathy is an ailment affecting the retina, leading to disturbed vision. It is sometimes a complication of diabetes mellitus.

A stye develops when infection occurs at the root of an eyelash.

HEARING

Your hearing system is concerned with sound, but it is also closely involved with your sense of balance. It lets your brain know of any changes in the position of your head, for example if it is tilting or turning round.

Your ear has three main parts: the outer ear, the middle ear and the inner ear. Your eardrum, a thin skin-like membrane, divides the outer from the middle ear.

Sound waves are collected and channelled by the outer ear on to your eardrum. That vibrates, passing the sound to your middle ear. There, the sounds are magnified by three small bones, while two small muscles absorb large vibrations to protect your inner ear from very loud noises. The magnified sound continues on to your inner ear and reaches the nerves of the cochlea. (Cochlea is the Latin word for snail shell, which is what it looks like.) The nerves transmit the sound signals to the hearing centres in your brain.

To keep an even pressure on both sides of your eardrum, air has to reach the middle ear. That is done through the eustachian tube connecting the inner ear to an area at the back of your nose and throat. The tube opens when you swallow or yawn to allow air to enter. The nerves of your middle ear that are concerned with balance get their signals from a fluid contained in three semicircular canals, or channels, in each ear. These are situated at right angles to each other to sense the dimensions of space. The fluid moves according to the position of your head. The nerve cells transmit the messages they receive to centres in the brain and to the spinal cord. That helps your body to adjust its balance.

Common ailments

Some hearing loss is not at all unusual in older people. If you have hearing changes, check with your doctor to see that nothing is wrong. Hearing is disturbed by anything that interferes with the travel of sound waves to the cochlea – for instance, too much wax in the outer ear, a perforated eardrum or a disease affecting the middle ear. Disease connected with the cochlea, or any of its nerve connections to the central nervous system, will also affect how well you hear.

Your sensitivity to sound may lose its sharpness, the older you are. The range of sounds you can hear lessens and the higher frequencies of someone else's speech may seem slightly muffled. The hearing centres in your brain may take longer to analyse and interpret the signals they receive.

Some medicines can upset your hearing system. Depending on which part of the system they act on – the nerve signals or the brain centre, for example – there may be some loss of hearing.

Tinnitus, a ringing noise in your ears, may also be a side-effect of some drugs, especially aspirin, although it can also occur for other reasons which are not fully understood.

Infection within the ear may also lead to hearing problems. Menière's disease is sometimes a result of infection or injury to the part of your ear that is concerned with balance. Sometimes its cause is unknown.

Otitis is inflammation of the ear, or a part of it.

SMELL AND TASTE

Your senses of smell and taste are closely linked. It can, for example, be difficult to distinguish between an apple and an onion if you have temporarily lost your sense of smell, which is the more sensitive of the two systems.

When you breathe in air containing odours, nerve endings deep in the nose are receptive to the particles that make different smells. The nerves then transmit the messages to the brain centres, which analyse and respond to the messages they receive.

Your taste buds are situated in projections on the tongue, called papillae. Taste buds, which are really specialised nerve endings, are also found in the membranes of part of the throat. These specialised nerve endings respond to four different sensations – sweetness, sourness, saltiness and bitterness. As with your other senses, the nerves signal to the brain centres which analyse the messages. But taste also depends on other messages the brain receives, such as sight and smell, and changes in temperature, pressure and texture on the membranes of your mouth and throat.

Common ailments

Partly because of the reduced speed at which your brain centres analyse the signals as you grow older, your senses of smell and taste are similarly reduced. Food may no longer seem as tasty or flowers smell as perfumed as they did when you were younger.

Nasal congestion (a stuffy nose) can result from infection, such as a cold, or it may be a side-effect of some medicines. It leads to a reduction in both your sense of smell and your sense of taste.

Nose bleeds may result from a knock, when tiny blood vessels are damaged. They can also result from ailments affecting your circulatory system, such as raised blood pressure.

Rhinitis is inflammation of the nose; sinusitis is inflammation affecting cavities (sinuses) in the cheekbones and above the eyes.

Nasal polyps are growths on the membranes in the nose. Polyps can appear on similar types of membrane in other parts of your body.

Black tongue occurs when the papillae on your tongue lengthen, and is not really an ailment. The colour and condition of your tongue can, however, tell your doctor a lot about your state of health.

What medicines do

A number of medicines for eye or ear ailments are dispensed in liquid form, to be used as drops. Because your senses are delicate systems, medicine containers and implements used to treat diseases should be especially clean. Eye-droppers should be used only for the length of time stated in the directions.

Medicines used for your eyes should be sterile (germ-free) and should not normally be kept for very long after they have been opened. Check with your doctor or pharmacist about when you should dispose of medicines. If you have been given eye-drops to use, ask your doctor how best to ensure that they reach the part of the eye that needs treatment. You should not treat ailments of your eyes and ears without first checking with your doctor or pharmacist.

There are several kinds of inflammation and infection of the eye and ear. Inflammation may be reduced by different types of drug, such as corticosteroids and antibiotics.

Analgesics

These pain relievers are used in some ear-drops.

Astringents

These are solutions that act on the surface of membranes to toughen them. Hamamelis (witch-hazel) is an astringent that is used in small amounts in some eye-drops, such as *Clearine, Optrex Eye Lotion, Optrex Eye Drops*.

Local anaesthetics

These block the pain signals of nerves around the area where they are applied. Benzocaine and lidocaine [lignocaine] are local anaesthetics sometimes included in remedies for sore throats. Products that contain local anaesthetics include: *AAA Spray, Bonjela pastilles, Rinstead gel, Strepsils spray, Tyrozets*, etc.

Oils

Almond oil and olive oil are among those used in products to soften ear wax. Oil-containing products include: *Earex Ear Drops*.

Sympathomimetics

These act on the blood vessels and nerves. Products that contain sympathomimetics include: *Otrivine*, used for nose problems; *Eye Dew* eye preparations. (For medicines used to treat infections, see: Your Defence Systems.)

Some other drugs and their brand names

Acetazolamide *Diamox*

This is a diuretic drug that may be used to reduce the pressure in your eye if you have glaucoma. Possible side-effects: headache, dizziness, drowsiness, lack of appetite, depression, rash, confusion.

Aluminium acetate

Inflammation of your outer ear may be treated with this astringent.

Docusate sodium *Molcer, Waxsol*, etc

This is used in ear-drops to soften ear wax.

Dorzolamide *Trusopt*

This may be used in eye-drops if you have glaucoma. Possible side-effects: bitter taste, feeling sick, headache, stinging in the eyes, blurred sight.

Hypromellose *Isopto Plain/Alkaline, Moisture-Eyes, Tears Naturale*, etc

This is used for dry eyes if you have tear deficiency.

Latanoprost *Xalatan*

This may be used in eye-drops if you have glaucoma. Possible side-effects: changes in the colour of your eyes, eye irritation.

Timolol maleate *Timoptol, Glaucol*, etc

This is a beta-blocker contained in eye-drops that may be used if you have glaucoma. You should not use this if you have asthma or heart failure, unless your doctor has agreed this with you. (See also 'Beta-blockers' on p 42 in: Your Heart and Blood Vessels.)

Pilocarpine hydrochloride *Isopto Carpine, Sno-Pilo*, etc

This reduces pressure in the eyes by contracting the pupil and allowing the aqueous fluid to drain. Eye-drops are used to treat glaucoma. Possible side-effects: reduced ability to see in poor light, headache, blurred vision.

Polyvinyl alcohol *Hypotears, Liquifilm Tears, Sno Tears*

This is used for dry eyes if you have tear deficiency.

Sodium bicarbonate ear-drops

This is used to soften ear wax.

Your Skin

You may not think of your skin as a 'system' of your body but it performs a great number of necessary functions carried out by no other system. It acts as protection. It provides insulation. It helps produce the body's supply of vitamin D. It guards against over-exposure to the sun. It contains the nerves for your sense of touch. It contains glands to keep you waterproof, to regulate your body temperature and to get rid of waste matter. Your skin is first to receive all the knocks of life.

The outer layer of skin is called the epidermis, which is made up of several layers of different kinds of cell. Epidermis cells gather in greater numbers where the skin is thickest, such as the palms of your hands and soles of your feet. The epidermis cells are constantly being shed and replaced by new ones from below. The outer layer of cells are not living, so they need no supply of blood for nourishment. As long as they remain unbroken, they prevent germs from getting into your system. The outer layer has a very thin covering of fatty sebum (oil) to keep it flexible.

The deeper layers of the epidermis contain a pigment called melanin. The more you have of that pigment, the browner your skin will be. It acts to protect you from the rays of the sun.

The inner layer of your skin, the dermis of true skin, is made up of connective tissue that is richly supplied with blood vessels, nerves and muscle.

The sensations of touch, pain, pressure, heat and cold are transmitted to the brain from the nerves in the skin. The nerve endings gather in their thousands. Some areas, such as your fingertips, have a greater concentration of nerve endings than comparatively insensitive areas such as your ear lobes.

Your skin's reaction to heat or cold leads to the blood vessels widening or narrowing. That causes more, or less, blood to flow through the skin, resulting in a greater or smaller loss of heat from your body.

Your temperature is also regulated by your skin through the sweat glands. They collect from the blood a fluid, sweat, that contains water, salt and waste matter. The fluid is deposited in pores on the surface of your skin. As the sweat evaporates, it cools the surface of your body. Sebaceous glands are also located in the skin, which produce oil to keep the skin waterproof and supple.

Hair and nails are really a type of skin. Your hair grows from roots set in pockets (follicles) in the dermis. The beds of your nails, like your hair roots, are in the dermis. The pink colour of your nails is due to their translucent quality, which allows the blood capillaries of the dermis to show through.

Common ailments

Skin reflects your general physical and emotional health, and this is why the doctor may have a good look at your skin, hair and nails. An ailment affecting one area of skin may also show up on another area some distance away. That is because your skin is really one large organ of your body. It covers such a wide area that it can be subject to a variety of problems.

Dermatitis is the medical name for an inflammation of the skin. Contact dermatitis occurs when your skin comes into contact with substances that irritate it or to which you are allergic.

Pruritus is itching skin; it has a number of causes, some unexplained. Dry skin may lead to an itching feeling. Skin cells flake all the time but dry skins may flake more as they shed the cells. Tension and stress can produce itching skin, as can an allergy. Itching skin may or may not be accompanied by a rash, which is spots of inflammation. Itching can, however, be a symptom of an underlying problem, such as a blood disorder.

Blushing is caused by a rush of blood to vessels on the face and neck. What seems like a permanent blush may be rosacea, a condition in which the blood capillaries have dilated (widened). An acne-like rash may also accompany that ailment. 'Liver spots' that may look like freckles commonly occur in later years, especially on the hands and face; they are harmless colourings.

Eczema is a general term for inflammation affecting mainly the top-most layer of the skin, the epidermis. Eczema may be dry and flaking or wet with weeping spots. Hives (urticaria) is a condition in which there are itching swellings on the skin. Hives, eczema and types of contact dermatitis can all be caused by allergies.

Dandruff occurs when the skin on the scalp flakes off as scales. It is often caused by a yeast micro-organism, a type of fungus, and it can cause itching. Scaling of the scalp can also be caused by a type of eczema.

Fungus infections can affect the nails. But nails that are too brittle, too soft, that are heavily ridged or that are speckled may be due to some other disorder of your body. A fungus infection of the skin may also cause athlete's foot.

Boils and carbuncles occur when germs gain entrance to the skin and cause pus to form. They may also be a symptom of other ailments.

Sores appear when skin is under pressure, perhaps through lying in only one position. The blood supply to tissues may be cut off, causing pressure sores. These can lead to the skin breaking, leaving the way open for infection to enter. Blisters occur if skin is constantly rubbed, or if it is burnt. Some infections can cause blisters. The watery fluid within blisters acts as protection while the skin tries to heal itself.

Warts (fleshy lumps) and callouses (hard lumps) may also occur on skin. These, too, have a number of causes.

Cancer is another ailment that can affect skin cells. In many cases, skin cancer can be caused by over-exposure to the harmful ultraviolet rays of the sun – ultraviolet A (UVA) and ultraviolet B (UVB). UVA rays generally do not cause sunburn but can contribute to long-term skin changes leading to cancer. UVB rays can cause sunburn and also contribute to the longer-term changes in the skin that can lead to cancer. Harmful rays can penetrate overcast skies, for example in hot climates, when skin can still be burnt.

What medicines do

Medicines used to prevent and treat skin diseases are supplied in various forms – creams, lotions, gels or powders, for example – that are applied directly to the skin. These are known as 'topical' medicines. Topical treatments also include certain shampoos that may be used to treat dandruff.

Other drugs used to treat skin ailments may be taken by mouth. Because skin is so sensitive, medicines used for skin ailments may produce unwanted reactions such as itching, rashes or allergies in different people. That is an important reason why you should not give any of your medicines, including creams, to a friend (see 'Sharing medicines', p 21).

Topical medicines used for skin ailments

ASTRINGENTS

These act on the surface of the skin to harden it. Zinc salts, aluminium salts and tannin derivatives such as hamamelis (witch-hazel) are the astringents most often used. Products containing astringents used for pain and inflammation include: *Sprilon spray, TCP Ointment, Vasogen.*

CREAMS AND OINTMENTS

Although these may seem similar, ointments are more greasy than creams. Petroleum jelly and liquid paraffin are often used in ointments. Wool fat (lanolin) may also be used even though it might cause reactions. Creams and ointments are used for various skin problems.

DUSTING POWDERS

These are used where areas of skin are in contact with each other, such as under the breasts. They help prevent friction. Dusting powders can cake and rub if they absorb moisture from very damp areas.

EMOLLIENTS

These smooth and soften the skin by oiling it. This is the function of most cosmetic creams. Applications may contain vegetable oils or animals fats such as wool fats (lanolin). Liquid paraffin, petroleum jellies, beeswax and urea may also be used in emollients. Emollient products include: *aqueous cream*, *Calmurid*, *Nutraplus*, *Ultrabase*.

LINIMENTS

These liquids may be analgesic (pain-relieving) or soothing, or they may stimulate the skin's reaction. They are often rubbed into the skin and the action of the massage may help relieve the ache or pain.

LOTIONS

These are used to apply drugs to the skin. They cool inflamed skin and are used when skin is unbroken. Shake lotions contain powders that leave a deposit on the skin after they have dried. They are used for scabbed and dried skin ailments. They may be used to relieve itching. Products of this type include: *Calamine lotion*.

PASTES

These preparations are stiffer than creams and ointments. They may be used to protect areas where skin is damaged or to apply drugs to scaly areas.

RUBEFACIENTS

These are used on the skin to cause blood vessels near the surface to dilate (widen). They produce a redness and warmth. That reaction is sometimes used to relieve pain that lies deeper in the skin, muscles or joints. Products having such effects may be called 'counter-irritants'. Methyl salicylate (wintergreen), camphor oil and menthol are among the drugs commonly used in skin preparations. Strong-smelling oils may also be added. Products of this type include: *Algipan*, *Menthol and Wintergreen Embrocation*, *oil of wintergreen*, *Radian-B*, *Ralgex* as a balm or spray, *Transvasin*.

SHAMPOOS

Shampoos that are used to control dandruff may contain a variety of substances, including mild detergents. Zinc pyrithione, selenium sulphide, coal tar and salicylic acid are all substances that may be in shampoos for dandruff. Shampoos containing one or more of these include: *Clinitar*, *Head & Shoulders*, *Ionil T*, *Polytar*, *Psoriderm*, etc.

SUNSCREENS

Sunscreen preparations contain substances that help protect the skin against the harmful rays of the sun – ultraviolet A (UVA) and ultraviolet B (UVB). The container normally carries information on how much protection the sunscreen aims to give against UVB rays: this is known as the sun protection factor (SPF). It indicates how much longer you can stay in the sun without burning, compared to how long you could stay if your skin were not protected. For example, if you can stay in the sun for 10 minutes without burning, a sunscreen with an SPF of 15 would allow you to stay in the sun fifteen times that, or 150 minutes (two and a half hours). Similarly, an SPF of 8 would allow you to stay 80 minutes (one hour 20 minutes). However, not all sunscreens protect you against both UVA and UVB rays – and over-exposure to both types of ray can in the long-term lead to skin cancers. (See 'Common ailments', p 108.)

Some other types of skin medicine

As well as being available in various forms, topical medicines may contain other drugs used to treat different types of ailment. Among the types of drug used are the following.

ANTIBIOTICS

These are drugs that are used to kill certain types of germ. When they are used as topical medicines, they deal only with organisms on the top layers of the skin. If the infection is deeper, into the dermis or true skin, they are often given by mouth. Some types of germ are becoming resistant to antibiotics, partly because of the over-use of such medicines. Some also cause rashes or other allergic reactions. (See also: Your Defence Systems.)

ANTIFUNGAL DRUGS

These are used to treat fungus infections. Clotrimazole, econazole nitrate, tolnaftate and the undecenoates are drugs often used in medicines to treat fungal infections. Products of this type include: *Canesten, Ecostatin, Mycota, Tinaderm, Tineafax.*

ANTIHISTAMINES

These act to block the skin's reaction to irritants. They can cause allergic reactions and should not be used for long periods. Antihistamines are also taken by mouth. Antazoline, diphenhydramine, mepyramine maleate and promethazine are antihistamines often incorporated in products for the skin. Such medicines include: *Anthisan, Caladryl, Wasp-Eze.*

ANTISEPTICS

Sometimes called germicides, these kill germs and prevent infection. Alcohols, cetrimide, chlorhexidine and hexachlorophane are among the antiseptics used. Medicines containing antiseptics include: *Cetavlex, Dermalex lotion, Dettol cream, TCP cream and liquid.*

CORTICOSTEROIDS

Also known as 'steroids', these suppress inflammation and allergic skin reactions. They relieve symptoms rather than provide a cure. They should be applied sparingly and not used over a long period, unless your doctor tells you otherwise. Because corticosteroids mask symptoms, untreated infections may spread. When you stop applying them the ailment may return worse than before. Their use on facial skin for anything more than a few days may cause permanent red veins (a condition called telangiectasia) because steroids can cause the skin to become thinner, especially in older people.

LOCAL ANAESTHETIC DRUGS

These act on the nervous system to deaden the skin's reaction to pain. They may produce allergic reactions, such as rashes. Benzocaine and lidocaine [lignocaine] are local anaesthetics often used in skin preparations. Products containing local anaesthetics include: *Anodesyn ointment and suppositories, BurnEze, Germoloids suppositories, xylocaine ointment* for use on haemorrhoids (piles), *Wasp-Eze spray. Dermidex* and *Lanacane* are used to calm itching and pain, for example around the anus (bottom) or private parts.

Some other drugs and their brand names

Betamethasone *Betnovate, Fucibet,* etc

A corticosteroid, this may be used to treat resistant eczema or other severe inflammatory disorders. Possible side-effects: spreading and worsening of untreated infections, thinning of skin.

Coal tar *Alphosyl, Carbo-Dome, Clinitar, Psoriderm,* etc

Psoriasis or eczema may be treated with this. It should not be used on broken skin. It stains skin, hair and clothes. Possible side-effects: skin irritation, rashes, skin sensitivity to light.

Clobetasol propionate *Dermovate*

A corticosteroid, this may be used for a short time to treat severe eczema and other severe inflammatory disorders. Possible side-effects: spread and worsening of untreated infections, thinning of skin.

Hydrocortisone *Dermacort, Dioderm, Efcortelan, Eurax HC, Hydrocortisyl, Lanacort,* etc

A corticosteroid, this may be used to treat mild inflammatory skin disorders, including eczema. It is also contained in some over-the-counter medicines (see 'What is a drug?', p 3) that you can buy to treat, for example, insect-bite reactions.

Ketoconazole *Nizoral, Nizoral Dandruff Shampoo, Neutrogena Long Lasting Dandruff Control,* etc

This is an anti-fungal drug that may be contained in shampoos or scalp creams. Some are available only on prescription. Possible side-effect: skin irritation.

Metronidazole *Metrogel,* etc

This is an antibacterial medicine. It may be contained in a cream used for rosacea, an ailment that affects the skin on your face. Possible side-effect: skin irritation.

Your Blood and Nutrition

Your blood

Like the 'middle-man' in the retail trade, blood acts as a supplier to your cells, tissues and organs. Using the transport system of your heart and blood vessels, your blood carries in it the nutrients and oxygen your body cells need for fuel. It also supplies areas of your body with products manufactured in other areas.

But blood is much more than a supply system. It carries hormones (chemical messengers) that help control your body's activities. It contains antibodies that are used in your defence system. It takes away the waste products of cells and tissues for disposal by the kidneys and skin, and the waste gas, carbon dioxide, for disposal through the breathing system.

More than half your blood is made up of plasma, a straw-coloured fluid that mostly consists of water. Just under half of your blood consists of blood cells. Plasma is important in regulating the balance of fluid in your body and is responsible for the consistency of your blood, that is whether it is thick or thin. Many important proteins are dissolved in the plasma. One, called fibrinogen, is made in the liver and is essential for the clotting process of your blood. Other proteins, formed in your lymph system, include the antibodies that you need to establish immunity to diseases and infections.

Proteins in blood plasma are constantly changing, depending on the amounts used by the rest of your cells and organs, and the amounts of protein stored in the body, especially by the liver. Among the other substances found in the plasma are sodium, potassium, calcium, chloride, bicarbonate, glucose, urea, uric acid and cholesterol. There are also small quantities of a wide variety of other materials.

Your blood cells are of three types – red corpuscles, white corpuscles and platelets. Red corpuscles carry oxygen to your tissues. White corpuscles act to defend your body from bacteria and irritants. Platelets are important to help your blood clot, for example to stop blood loss from a wound.

Red blood cells are formed in the red marrow of some bones, such as your ribs and pelvis and the ends of long bones such as those in your legs. Red cells contain essential products such as iron and vitamins. Damaged and old red cells are removed by the spleen, a firm organ that lies just below the diaphragm near the stomach. The spleen retains iron from broken-down red cells for use in fresh cells. Iron is, however, also stored in your liver.

White blood cells are your body's main defence against infections. These cells can multiply rapidly and travel quickly to an affected area of your body. They surround and kill the bacteria causing the infection. White blood cells are formed from cells originating in bone marrow. The lymph system, your thymus gland and your spleen are concerned with the production of these defence cells. Pus is a mixture of dead white cells and the bacteria they are trying to eliminate.

Nutrition

Nutrition is concerned with what you eat, the way your body converts what you eat and how your body uses the converted substances. Good nutrition depends on five things:

1 Eating the food that is right for you.
2 Your body converting the nutrients into simpler substances.
3 Your body absorbing these substances.
4 Your body making enough of the nutrients it can manufacture.
5 Your cells, tissues and organs using the nutrients for energy, body maintenance and growth.

The foods you must have are proteins, vitamins, minerals, fats and carbohydrates (starches and sugars). Your body can manufacture sugars from fats. It can manufacture fats from sugars and proteins, according to its needs. It cannot manufacture proteins from sugars and fats.

Essential substances, called amino acids, are contained in proteins, which are needed for growth and for replacing the tissue proteins that are constantly being broken down.

Vitamins help transform other food substances into necessary parts of bones, skin, glands, nerves, brain and blood. Vitamins are required in only relatively small amounts. However, if you do not have them in your diet, or if your body fails to absorb them properly, you can suffer from deficiency problems. Vitamins are known by letters – A, B, C, D, E and K, for example. In some groups there may be more vitamin types, such as vitamins B_1 and B_{12}.

There are probably at least twenty minerals used by your body, many of which are essential to health. Among them are sodium, potassium, iron, magnesium and phosphorus. You need traces of zinc and copper. Iodide, chloride and fluoride are also necessary elements. The minerals make up the body salts.

Food is also important as a source of energy. Simple carbohydrates such as sugars contribute only energy; excess energy may be stored as fat, making the person overweight.

The level of food substances the body needs changes as you mature and develop. Older people's requirements differ from those of children and teenagers, for example. Your needs also change as a result of ailments or disease.

Common ailments

Anaemia is possibly the most well-known problem affecting the blood, and it can affect people of all ages. Anaemia is not a disease in itself; rather it is a symptom of a number of different diseases or disorders. Anaemia is a reduction, below normal, of the number, quality or proportion of the red oxygen-carrying cells in your blood. It may be due to loss of blood, perhaps steadily over a period of time from such ailments as bleeding ulcers, haemorrhoids (piles) or a hiatus hernia. A poor diet, resulting in you not getting enough of the essential proteins, vitamins and minerals you need, can contribute to anaemia. It may be due to diseases of the bone marrow or be a side-effect of some drugs. Under-activity of your thyroid gland and other illnesses such as kidney failure may also cause anaemia.

Anaemia can also be the result of your body failing to absorb certain food nutrients. That may stem from ailments somewhere within your digestive system. A serious form of anaemia, called pernicious anaemia, may arise as a result of your body failing to produce a substance needed to help you absorb vitamin B_{12}.

For these reasons, two people, both with anaemia but coming about in different ways, can receive widely differing treatments from their doctors.

Deficiency disease, when you lack one or more of the essential proteins, vitamins or minerals, can also be due to a number of ailments. Malnutrition may be one cause. That is not, as some people think, a lack of food. It is a lack of the right food. Malnutrition can lead to you being over-weight, just as much as it contributes to under-weight.

Deficiency disorders can also be a side-effect of some drugs needed to treat other ailments. A loss of potassium, for example, may be due to the actions of a diuretic drug taken for raised blood pressure.

Ailments affecting any of the blood-making organs – bone-marrow, lymph system or spleen – may also lead to blood disorders. Leukaemia is the name given to several types of cancer affecting cells in these organs. That, in turn, affects your white blood cells. A cancerous tumour in your lymph system will also affect the quality of your white blood cells and some plasma cells.

What medicines do

Many of the drugs used to treat disorders of the blood are aimed at replacing or supplementing the body's blood supply. They should be taken like any other medicine, according to your doctor's or pharmacist's advice. (See also 'Sustained-release drugs', p 54).

Calcium salts

These may be used if you have problems absorbing calcium from your food, or to help strengthen your bones. An excessive intake of calcium salts can cause stomach upsets, feeling sick, constipation, palpitations and kidney damage. Medicines containing calcium include: *Calciohew, calcium gluconate tablets, Sandocal*, etc.

Iron salts

In some types of anaemia these may be used. Possible side-effects include: feeling sick, stomach upsets, constipation or diarrhoea, dark-coloured stools. Iron-containing medicines include: *Feospan, Ferrocontin Continus, Ferrograd, ferrous fumarate, ferrous gluconate, ferrous glycine sulphate, ferrous sulphate, Fersaday, Fersamal, Galfer, Niferex-150, Plesmet, Slow-Fe.*

Oral rehydration salts

These are discussed on page 35 in: Your Digestive System.

Potassium salts

These may be used to supplement your diet or to replace potassium lost through the action of other drugs, such as diuretics or anti-arrhythmic drugs. Possible side-effects: feeling sick, bowel problems. It is important to swallow tablets with plenty of water so that they go down properly. Medicines containing potassium include: *Kay-Cee-L, Kloref, Nu-K, Sando-K.*

Vitamins

It should be remembered that vitamins are medicines. If you intend to buy vitamin tablets, or the so-called 'tonics' that may contain vitamins, you should check with your doctor whether you need to take them. Most people can get all the vitamins they need by normal healthy eating. A number of vitamin preparations available, for example, in health food shops, may contain a dose that can be harmful to you. You should check with your pharmacist that any vitamin preparations will not interfere with medicines you already take. Vitamin C is the most common vitamin that might be needed by older people, and vitamin D for those who get too little sun and have a poor diet.

MULTIVITAMINS

With some deficiency problems, your doctor may prescribe tablets or syrup containing more than one vitamin, such as 'vitamin capsules'. However, there are many preparations – tablets, capsules, elixirs, syrups – that contain several vitamins, many of which may be unnecessary for you. Some may also contain calcium or iron. Check with your doctor or pharmacist.

VITAMIN A

Vitamin A is found naturally in such foods as liver, fish-liver oils, eggs, milk and dairy products, green vegetables, and fruits and vegetables such as carrots, peaches and tomatoes. A normal healthy diet will usually provide all that you need. In rare cases, extra amounts may be needed by people with some stomach and bowel diseases. An excess of vitamin A can cause: headache, feeling sick, diarrhoea, rough skin, dry hair and liver damage. Medicines containing vitamin A include: *halibut-liver oil capsules* and many multivitamin preparations.

VITAMIN B$_1$ (THIAMIN)

Vitamin B$_1$ is found naturally in such foods as bran, wholemeal bread, brown rice, pasta, pulses (lentils, etc), meat, fish, nuts, eggs and vegetables. A normal healthy diet will usually provide all that you need. In rare cases, extra amounts may be needed if you have an over-active thyroid, or if you have some disease of the liver or intestine, or if you have problems of alcoholism. An excess of thiamin can affect your body's ability to absorb other vitamins. Medicines containing vitamin B$_1$ include: *Becosym*, *Benerva*, *Compound Vitamin B tablets* and many multivitamin supplements.

VITAMIN B₁₂

Vitamin B_{12} is found naturally in such foods as liver, most animal products, and seaweed. A normal healthy diet will usually provide all that you need. People who eat mostly refined or processed foods sometimes may need extra vitamin B_{12}. Strict vegetarians or vegans may also need extra vitamin B_{12}. Medicines containing vitamin B_{12} include: *Compound Vitamin B tablets, Becosym, Vigranon B* and many multivitamin preparations.

VITAMIN C

Vitamin C is found naturally in most fresh fruit and vegetables, including leafy green vegetables. Both fruit and vegetables lose some vitamin C if they are cooked. A normal healthy diet will usually provide all that you need. People suffering from iron-deficiency anaemia may need extra vitamin C because it helps iron absorption. Some older people may need extra vitamin C if they are not getting enough through their usual diet. An excess of vitamin C may cause diarrhoea or stomach upsets, or bring on an attack of gout. Medicines containing vitamin C include: *ascorbic acid tablets, Redoxon* and many multivitamin preparations.

VITAMIN D

Vitamin D is contained naturally in such foods as milk, dairy products, egg yolks and oily fish (sardines, tuna, salmon). It is also made by the body as the result of sunlight on the skin. You may be prescribed vitamin D if you do not get enough sun or if you suffer from osteomalacia, a type of bone weakness in adults. You may also be given vitamin D because of problems of fat absorption. An excess of vitamin D may cause loss of appetite, feeling sick, diarrhoea, sweating, headache, thirst, weariness. Medicines containing vitamin D include: *Abidec, Alfa D, Cacit D3, Calcichew, calciferol tablets, Rocaltrol* and many multivitamin preparations.

VITAMIN E

Vitamin E is found naturally in vegetable oils, green leafy vegetables and wholemeal cereals. A normal healthy diet will usually provide all that you need. You may be prescribed this if you have problems of absorption. An excess of vitamin E may cause stomach upsets, feeling sick, diarrhoea. Medicines containing vitamin E include: *Ephynal* and many multivitamin preparations.

Vitamin K

Vitamin K is found naturally in milk, yoghurt and green leafy vegetables. The body also manufactures it in the intestine. A normal healthy diet will usually provide all that you need. However, you may be prescribed vitamin K if you have certain stomach or bowel diseases or have been taking some anticoagulant drugs. Medicines containing vitamin K include: *menadiol sodium phosphate tablets*, *Konakion* and many multivitamin preparations.

Tonics

So-called tonics, or 'pick-me ups', generally have little therapeutic (healing) effect, other than psychological; that is, you think they will do you good. If you feel you need a tonic, perhaps because you feel tired or run down, check with your doctor to see if anything is wrong. If you need a medicine, your doctor will advise you what to take.

Your Defence Systems

When it is attacked, by injury or disease for example, your body acts to defend itself. It can muster an army of cells to fight back and to build barriers to keep the damage from spreading. The body can also build up defences so that it is prepared if disease strikes.

There are many would-be attackers. They include bacteria, viruses, toxins (poisons), fungi and minute organisms called protozoa.

Bone marrow, your lymph system, liver, spleen and blood cells are all involved in defending you. They also call on other organs and systems to help.

Infection

Infection or injury can affect any part of you. Depending on the nature of the problem, the body will respond in a number of stages. Tissues that are injured release a chemical substance that sets up a protective response by your body. Blood vessels dilate (widen) so that there is an increased blood flow to the area. That is the meaning of 'inflammation', for the tissues swell, look red and feel warmer.

The blood brings with it white blood cells that gather in large numbers. They surround and try to destroy the cause of the inflammation. Body fluids gather at the injured site, bringing with them more white blood cells and immune bodies. These also help in the removal of dead bacteria, destroyed tissue cells and blood cells. When the invader has been eliminated, your body can set about repairing itself.

Immunity

Your immune system is essentially concerned with your body's ability to recognise and dispose of a substance that it sees as being harmful. When it detects foreign substances, your immune system goes into action to protect your tissues and cells.

The response of your immune system can be broadly divided into two categories. There is the immune action that takes place in the body fluids. There is also the action that aims to contain, or limit, cells that it recognises as being foreign and harmful.

When a foreign substance is detected, antibodies are released into the body fluids from plasma cells. An antibody, or a group of antibodies, is designed to attack a specific target, such as one type of virus or a type of bacteria. Its targets are called antigens. 'Memory' cells remain in your lymph system and stand ready for any future encounters with antigens.

The part of your immune system that deals with cell activity is mainly concerned with a delayed response. Examples of that type of response include: defence against slowly developing bacterial disease affecting cells; rejecting transplanted organs; getting rid of body cells that are infected with viruses; or attacking cells affected by cancerous growths. In such cases white blood cells set about destroying the invader, either directly or by releasing chemicals to stimulate body action. This process enhances the effectiveness of the immune system's activities.

Immunity can be gained in several ways. You may be born with it, a natural inheritance passed on from parents. That is called passive immunity. Immunity may come about through contact with someone else with the disease, to which your body responds. You can acquire immunity through having the disease yourself, so that the next time the virus or bacterium is around, your body is prepared. Through vaccines containing bacteria or viruses that have been killed or tamed, you can be given a mild version of the disease. That encourages your body to build up antibodies without the need to have the full disease. Or you can be given, by injection, ready-made antibodies that have been produced elsewhere, the so-called passive immunity which lasts only for a period of time.

Common ailments

Infections and diseases, whatever their cause, can be caught in a number of ways. However, there are six links necessary before the circle of infection can occur:

1 There must be a 'cause' – a virus, bacterium, etc.
2 It must have a 'home' in which to thrive and multiply. That may be in your body, in waste matter, in the ground, or in contaminated food or water.
3 It must have a way of leaving its 'home', for example on your breath or in waste matter.
4 It must have a way of transferring to a new 'home'. That may be in the air, carried by humans, animals or insects, or it can travel in drops of moisture, as in a sneeze.
5 It must have a way of entering its new 'home', such as through a wound or by being breathed in.
6 The host must be susceptible to the infection, either by having no immunity or by having insufficient resistance to it.

Lowered resistance can be caused by poor general health. It may stem from a poor diet and lack of the necessary nutrients needed to build up defences. It can be caused by one disease taking hold and providing a suitable environment for the spread of infection, such as bronchitis opening the door to pneumonia. Fever is an abnormally high temperature that may accompany infection.

Infectious diseases may be transmitted by several means – air, animals, water, food, contaminated objects, etc. Contagious diseases are passed from person to person by touch or contact. Many illnesses throughout the body are caused by infections of one sort or another.

Problems with the immune system can also lead to a variety of diseases.

Immuno-depression is an absence or deficient supply of the cells needed for your defences to work. It may be because of ailments affecting parts of the body, such as the thymus gland, blood or bone marrow, that help produce immune cells. It may be due to malnutrition, not eating enough of the essential nutrients. Or it may be caused by cancers, burns or viral infections overwhelming the system. AIDS (acquired immune deficiency syndrome) is an ailment that depresses the immune system.

Sometimes the immune system is deliberately lowered, for example if you have an organ or tissue transplant, to reduce the chances of your body rejecting the transplant.

Over-sensitivity occurs when the immune system over-reacts to the presence of foreign bodies. Hay fever, allergies and some types of asthma are the sorts of ailment that can result.

Auto-immune diseases happen as a result of the body failing to tolerate its own cells and tissues. For some reason, in such cases the body identifies its own cells and tissues as enemies and reacts to destroy them. Among the disorders in which this may happen are rheumatoid arthritis, some types of anaemia and some thyroid conditions.

Multiple myeloma, an excess of blood plasma cells, happens when the immune system over-produces antibodies and immunoglobulin, which is a protein that acts as an antibody.

Tumours and cancers

Cancer is a name given to many different body cell diseases. Normally, worn-out or damaged body cells are replaced by new cells; when there are enough of them, they stop forming. For example, new cells grow to repair tissue damage, and stop growing when the area is healed. In these cases, the cell growth is regulated. Sometimes, however, cell growth is not regulated. Cells continue to multiply until they form a mass of tissue known as a tumour. Tumours vary in size. Some remain small and are not worth removing. Others grow large enough to obstruct, or block, the proper function of other vessels and organs, and so they have to be removed. These sorts of tumour are known as benign, because the cells are normal and obey the rules.

Malignant tumours, or cancers, invade organs and tissues, robbing them of their food and blood supply and growing in a disorderly fashion. Unlike benign tumours, cancerous tumours can spread. They may invade tissues nearby. They may travel in the lymph system to set up roots elsewhere, or they may travel in the bloodstream. Many cancers can be cured if caught early enough but medical examination is needed to decide which tumours are benign and which are malignant.

What medicines do

Infection may be caused by any number of micro-organisms. As a result, the drugs used to prevent or treat infections depend mainly on which organism is, or is likely to be, responsible. As doctors and scientists identify more of the organisms causing infections, so they continually research and produce more drugs to fight them.

'Antibiotic' is the name popularly used for the drugs used to treat infections. Correctly speaking, antibiotics are medicines that are used to fight bacteria. When the organism is a virus, an antiviral drug is used; when it is a fungus, an antifungal is used, and so on.

In their fight for survival, organisms causing infection can become resistant to some antibiotics. Scientists and doctors have become concerned that, with the widespread use of antibiotics, more bacteria are becoming resistant to more drugs. Doctors have therefore been asked to try to use antibiotics only when they are likely to be most effective, and not to prescribe them 'just in case'. It is also why you should not expect to receive an antibiotic for illnesses not caused by bacteria – such as a cold or 'flu caused by a virus – unless you also have a bacterial infection with it.

Bacterial resistance is also one of the reasons why, if you are prescribed an antibiotic, you should complete the course. Do not stop just because the ailment seems to have cleared up. Unless it is killed completely, the micro-organism causing the infection may lurk to await another chance to strike, and next time it might have developed a better resistance to that medicine.

Allergy to drugs used to treat infections

Some people are over-sensitive (allergic) to some groups of antibiotic – such as penicillin or penicillin-like drugs. If you are allergic to such drugs, you should tell your doctor, so that he or she can suggest an antibiotic from another group. Side-effects such as rashes, a fever or joint pains may mean that you are allergic to the antibiotic. If you experience such effects, you should tell your doctor as soon as possible so that he or she can help you decide if that is the right medicine for you. Other side-effects can include stomach upsets or diarrhoea.

Groups of drugs that treat infection

Aminoglycosides are a group of drugs used for infections caused by bacteria. They include: gentamicin, neomycin, tobramycin, which may be contained in ear-drops or eye-drops.

Anthelmintics are used for infections caused by worms and similar organisms. They include mebendazole (*Ovex*) and piperazine (*Pripsen*).

Antibacterials are used for infections caused by bacteria. They include aminoglycosides, cephalosporins, penicillins, sulphonamides and tetracyclines (see under each heading in this section).

Antifungals may be used for infections caused by a fungus. They include ketoconazole, which may be used in anti-dandruff shampoos or lotions (see: Your Skin).

Antiseptics are used to kill or prevent the growth of organisms on the surface of the body (eg the skin). A number of different chemicals are used as antiseptics in creams, lotions and ointments. They are sometimes combined with disinfectants (see below).

Antiprotozoals are used for infections caused by protozoa such as malaria. Antimalaria medicines should generally be started one to two weeks before you travel and continued for at least four weeks after you return. They include chloroquine (*Avloclor*, *Nivaquine*, etc), mefloquine (*Larium*, etc), pyrimethamine with dapsone (*Maloprim*) and proguanil hydrochloride (*Paludrine*). Possible side-effects include: feeling sick, headache, sickness, dizziness, sleepiness, disturbed sleep, palpitations, tinnitus (ringing in your ears), rashes, itching, hair loss, sight disturbances.

Antivirals are used for infections caused by a virus. They include aciclovir, famciclovir, idoxuridine.

Cephalosporins are a group of drugs used against infections caused by bacteria. Some people who are allergic to penicillin and penicillin-like medicines may also be allergic to drugs of this group. They include cefaclor and cefuroxime. Possible allergic reactions: rashes, itching, hives (nettle rash), fever, joint pains.

Disinfectants are chemicals that reduce micro-organisms to harmless levels, although they may not destroy all micro-organisms. (See also 'Antiseptics', above.)

Penicillins are a group of drugs used to fight bacterial infections. They include amoxicillin [amoxycillin], ampicillin and flucloxacillin. Some people are allergic to penicillins and penicillin-like medicines: if you are allergic to one of them, you will be allergic to them all. If you get a skin rash, you should stop taking these medicines and tell your doctor immediately. He or she may then suggest another antibacterial to which you are not allergic.

Sulphonamides are a group of drugs used against infections caused by bacteria. They include co-trimoxazole, sulphacetamide and sulfa-salazine [sulphasalazine]. Possible side-effects: feeling sick, sickness, headache, reduced appetite, rashes, blood disorders, fever.

Tetracyclines are a group of drugs used against bacterial infections. They include doxycycline and oxytetracycline. Possible side-effects: feeling sick, diarrhoea.

Some drugs and their brand names

Aciclovir *Zovirax*

This antiviral may be used if you have shingles. Possible side-effects: skin rash, stomach upsets, headache, dizziness, feeling of tiredness.

Amoxicillin [amoxycillin] *Amix, Amoram, Amoxil*, etc

This antibacterial medicine may be used if you have bronchitis, ear infections or infections in your urinary system. It may also be used, together with other anti-ulcer drugs, if you have peptic ulcers (see also: Your Digestive System). Possible side-effects: feeling sick, diarrhoea, allergy (see also 'Penicillins', above).

Ampicillin *Penbritin*, etc

This antibacterial medicine may be used to treat respiratory infections and those of the ear, nose or throat. Possible side-effects: stomach upsets, allergy (see also 'Penicillins', p 129).

Cefaclor *Distaclor*

This is one of the cephalosporin group of medicines. Possible side-effects: headache, stomach upsets, feeling sick, dizziness, confusion, sleep disturbances, allergy (see also 'Cephalosporins', p 129).

Cefuroxime *Zinnat*

This is one of the cephalosporin group of medicines. It may be used if you have a chest infection, or infection of the urinary tract. Possible side-effects: headache, stomach upsets, feeling sick, dizziness, confusion, sleep disturbances, allergy (see also 'Cephalosporins', p 129).

Cephalexin *Ceporex, Keflex, Tenkorex*

This is one of the cephalosporin group of medicines. Possible side-effects: headache, stomach upsets, feeling sick, dizziness, confusion, sleep disturbances, allergy (see also 'Cephalosporins', p 129).

Chloramphenicol *Chloromycetin, Sno-Phenicol*

Ear-drops and eye-drops may contain this antibacterial. Possible side-effects: some people may be sensitive.

Clarithromycin *Klaricid*

This antibacterial medicine may be used, together with other anti-ulcer drugs, if you have peptic ulcers (see also: Your Digestive System). Possible side-effects: stomach upsets, feeling sick, headache, rash.

Co-amoxyclav *Augmentin*

This antibacterial medicine may be used to treat a wide range of infections. Possible side-effects: feeling sick, diarrhoea, allergy (see also 'Penicillins', p 129).

Co-trimoxazole *Bactrim, Septrin,* etc

This is a sulphonamide that may be used if you have bronchitis or a urinary infection. Possible side-effects: feeling sick, skin rash, diarrhoea, headache, sore tongue, tinnitus (ringing in your ears), jaundice (see also 'Sulphonamides', p 129).

Doxycycline *Doxylar, Vibramycin,* etc

This is one of the tetracyline group of medicines used to fight bacteria. Possible side-effects: feeling sick, diarrhoea, headache, sight disturbances, stomach pain.

Erythromycin *Erycen, Erymax, Erythrocin, Erythromid, Ilosone,* etc

This may be used in drops or ointment for eye or ear infections. Possible side-effects: feeling sick, sickness, diarrhoea, skin rash.

Famciclovir *Famvir*

This antiviral may be used if you have shingles. Possible side-effects: feeling sick, headache.

Flucloxacillin *Floxapen, Ladropen, Stafoxil,* etc

This is an antibacterial medicine. Possible side-effects: itchy rash, high temperature, joint pains (see also 'Penicillins', p 129).

Gentamicin *Cidomycin Topical, Garamycin, Genticin,* etc

This aminoglycoside may be contained in some anti-infective skin creams. Cream or ointment may be used if you have a bacterial infection of your skin. It may be used in drops or ointment for eye or ear infections.

Griseofulvin *Fulcin, Grisovin*

This is an antifungal medicine that may be used for scalp and nail infections. Possible side-effects: headache, feeling sick, sickness, skin rash, dizziness, tiredness. It may affect your ability to drive. Men should not father a child within six months of being treated with this.

Metronidazole *Flagyl, Rozex, Zadstat,* etc

This is an antibacterial medicine. Among other things, it may be used for infections including some leg ulcers, gum disease and dental infections. Tablets may also be used, together with other anti-ulcer drugs, if you have peptic ulcers (see also: Your Digestive System). Possible side-effects: feeling sick, sickness, unpleasant taste, stomach upsets, skin rash, drowsiness, dizziness, dark-coloured urine. You should not take alcohol if you are taking this medicine.

Miconazole *Daktarin* (as gel, cream, dusting powder or spray)

This may be used to treat fungal infections of your skin. Possible side-effects: skin irritation.

Neomycin sulphate *Betnesol-N, Neo-Cortef, Predsol-N,* etc

This is an aminoglycoside and may be used in ear- or eye-drops.

Oxytetracycline *Berkmycen, Oxymycin, Terramycin,* etc

This antibacterial may be used if you have chronic bronchitis, or if you have rosacea (see: Your Skin). Possible side-effects: feeling sick, sickness, diarrhoea, headache, sight disturbances, stomach pains (see also 'Tetracyclines', p 129).

Penicillin V [phenoxymethylpenicillin] *Apsin,* etc

This antibacterial may be used if you have tonsillitis or a throat infection. Possible side-effects: feeling sick, diarrhoea, rash, joint pains (see also 'Penicillins', p 129).

Pivampicillin *Pondocillin,* etc

This is a type of penicillin that may be used for a wide variety of infections. Possible side-effects: feeling sick, diarrhoea (see also 'Penicillins', p 129).

Tetracycline *Achromycin, Sustamycin, Tetrachel,* etc

This antibacterial may be used for a wide variety of infections. It may also be used, together with anti-ulcer drugs, if you have peptic ulcers (see also: Your Digestive System). Possible side-effects: feeling sick, diarrhoea, headache, sight disturbances (see also 'Tetracyclines', p 129).

Trimethoprim *Ipral, Monotrim, Trimopan,* etc

This is an antibacterial medicine that may be used if you have bronchitis or a urinary infection. Possible side-effects: stomach upsets, feeling sick, itching, skin rash.

Vaccines to prevent infection

Vaccines are among the medicines (prophylactics) used to prevent you catching an infection. That can be done by giving you a mild version of the disease to allow your system to build up antibodies to it. Or you may be given protection in the form of ready-made antibodies. Depending on the vaccine you may get no apparent reaction; or you may have a raised temperature or headache, or inflammation where you have had the injection. Your doctor will advise you whether there are any ailments against which you ought to seek protection at home or abroad.

Some of the diseases against which you might seek protection in the UK are: influenza ('flu), pneumonia and tetanus. Vaccinations against 'flu and pneumococcal infections (pneumonia) are likely to be especially recommended if you have diabetes, or a lung, heart or kidney disorder, or if you live in a residential home. If your spleen has been removed, or is not working properly, pneumococcal vaccination may be advised. Tetanus vaccination may also be recommended, especially for gardeners.

Other protection against infection

If you are going abroad, you might be advised to seek protection against any or all of the following: typhoid, tetanus, malaria, polio, hepatitis. What you might need will depend on the country you intend to visit and what you intend to do there. Because the malaria parasite has developed resistance to different antimalarial drugs – and which drug depends on which area – the medicines recommended may differ according to the part of the world you intend to go to, or you may be advised to take more than one type of tablet.

If you intend to go abroad, ask your doctor about the precautions at least three months in advance. Not all prophylactic medicines and vaccines are available free on the NHS: this applies especially to travel medicines, such as antimalaria tablets. (See also the entry for Medical Advisory Service for Travellers Abroad (Masta) in 'Useful Addresses'.)

Anti-cancer drugs

The drugs used in the treatment of some types of cancer are generally given in hospital, or at home under medical supervision, and are therefore not included in this book. Although most people receive them in hospital, they often go home between treatments. Some of the complex medicines used have unpleasant side-effects. The doctor should tell you what you might expect. A number of the medicines may also affect your body's response to dealing with infection, so you may be advised to take special care to avoid infections. Check with the doctor. (See also 'Tumours and cancers', p 126.)

Medicines for AIDS

As with cancers, medicines used in the fight against acquired immune deficiency syndrome (AIDS) are generally given under medical supervision in hospital and are, similarly, not included in this book. Some of these medicines have unpleasant side-effects and your doctor should tell you what you might expect.

Section 3
FURTHER INFORMATION

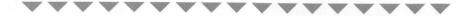

Useful Addresses

Alzheimer's Disease Society

Gordon House
10 Greencoat Place
London SW1P 1PH
Tel: 0171-306 0606
Fax: 0171-306 0808

Information, support and advice about caring for someone with Alzheimer's disease.

Arthritis Care

18 Stephenson Way
London NW1 2HD
Tel: 0171-916 1500
Helpline: 0800 289 170 (Mon to Fri, noon–4.00pm)

Information and support about living with arthritis.

British Association of Cancer United Patients (BACUP)

3 Bath Place
Rivington Street
London EC2A 3JR
Tel: 0171-696 9003 (booklets)
     0171-613 2121 (advice)
     0171-696 9000 (counselling)
Fax: 0171-696 9002
Freephone advice line for people outside London: 0800 181 199.

Support and information for cancer sufferers and their families.

British Dental Health Foundation

Eastlands Court
St Peter's Road
Rugby
Warwicks CV21 3QP
Helpline: 01788 546365

Information, advice and assistance on dental health and dental problems.

British Diabetic Association

10 Queen Anne Street
London W1M 0BD
Tel: 0171-323 1531
Fax: 0171-637 3644
Helpline: 0171-636 6112 (Mon to Fri, 9.00am–5.00pm)

Information and advice about living with diabetes.

British Heart Foundation

14 Fitzhardinge Street
London W1H 4DH
Tel: 0171-935 0185
Fax: 0171-486 5820

Information and advice about living with a heart problem.

British Homoeopathic Association

27A Devonshire Street
London W1N 1RJ
Tel: 0171-935 2163

List of medically qualified practitioners, pharmacies, manufacturers.

Cancerlink

11–21 Northdown Street
London N1 9BN
Tel: 0171-833 2451

Support and information for people with cancer and their families.

Chest, Heart and Stroke Scotland

65 North Castle Street
Edinburgh EH2 3LT
Tel: 0131-225 6963
Helpline: 0345 720 720 (Mon to Fri, 9.30am–4.00pm)

Literature, information and advice on dealing with chest, heart and stroke problems.

Continence Foundation

2 Doughty Street
London WC1N 2PH
Helpline: 0191-213 0050

Information and advice on continence problems.

Council for Involuntary Tranquilliser Addiction

Cavendish House
Brighton Road
Waterloo
Liverpool LL22 5NG
Helpline: 0151-949 0102

Information and advice about withdrawal, and support through withdrawal.

Drinkline

Petersham House
57A Hatton Garden
London EC1N 8HP
Freephone: 0500 801 802 (recorded information)
Helpline: 0345 32 02 02
Asianline: 0990 133480 (24-hour dial and listen – Hindi, Urdu, Gujerati)

National helpline for information, help and advice about drinking, including people worried about someone else's drinking.

Health Information Service

Freephone: 0800 66 55 44

*NHS helpline, government-funded. Information about health author-
ities, hospitals, waiting times, illnesses, services, support groups and
voluntary organisations.*

Hospital for Tropical Diseases Travel Clinic

Helpline: 0839 337 733 (premium rates)

Information and advice on travel immunisation.

Medical Advisory Service for Travellers Abroad (Masta)

Helpline: 0891 224 100 (24-hour line; premium rates)

Information and advice on travel immunisation.

National Drugs Helpline

Freephone: 0800 77 66 00

*Government-funded. Provides advice, information, counselling to
people who have a drug problem or are worried about someone with
a drug problem, whether with legal or illegal drugs. Literature for parents and grandparents concerned about young people.*

National Eczema Society

163 Eversholt Street
London NW1 1BU
Tel: 0171-388 4097

Advice and information on eczema and other skin diseases.

National Osteoporosis Society

PO Box 10
Radstock
Bath BA3 3YB
Tel: 01761 471771
Fax: 01761 471104
Helpline: 01761 472721

Information, literature and advice.

Northern Ireland Chest, Heart and Stroke Association

21 Dublin Road
Belfast BT2 7FJ
Tel: 01232 320184

Information on chest, heart and stroke problems.

Parkinson's Disease Society

22 Upper Woburn Place
London WC1H 0RA
Tel: 0171-383 3513
Fax: 0171-383 5754
Helpline: 0171-388 5798 (Mon to Fri 10.00am–4.00pm)

Information on Parkinson's disease.

Quit

Victory House
170 Tottenham Court Road
London W1P 0HA
Freephone: 0800 00 22 00

Telephone helpline, information and counselling on giving up smoking.

Standing Conference on Drug Abuse (SCODA)

32–36 Loman Street
London SE1 0EE
Tel: 0171-928 9500

National organisation for drug services. Provides information and guidance to professionals in education, prevention, treatment and care.

Stroke Association

123–127 Whitecross Street
London EC1Y 8JJ
Tel: 0171-490 7999

Information and advice about stroke.

About Age Concern

Know Your Medicines is one of a wide range of publications produced by Age Concern England, the National Council on Ageing. Age Concern England is actively engaged in training, information provision, fund raising and campaigning for retired people and those who work with them, and also in the provision of products and services such as insurance for older people.

A network of more than 1,400 local Age Concern groups, with the support of around 250,000 volunteers, aims to improve the quality of life for older people and develop services appropriate to local needs and resources. These include advice and information, day care, visiting services, transport schemes, clubs, and specialist facilities for older people who are physically and mentally frail.

Age Concern England is a registered charity dependent on public support for the continuation and development of its work.

Age Concern England
1268 London Road
London SW16 4ER
Tel: 0181-679 8000

Age Concern Scotland
113 Rose Street
Edinburgh EH2 3DT
Tel: 0131-220 3345

Age Concern Cymru
4th Floor
1 Cathedral Road
Cardiff CF1 9SD
Tel: 01222 371566

Age Concern Northern Ireland
3 Lower Crescent
Belfast BT7 1NR
Tel: 01232 245729

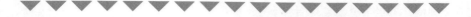

Publications from Age Concern Books

HEALTH AND CARE

The Community Care Handbook: The reformed system explained
Barbara Meredith

Written by one of the country's leading experts, the second edition of this hugely successful handbook provides a comprehensive overview of the first two years of implementation of the community care reforms and examines how the system has evolved. Containing extensive background information on the origins of the new system, this edition describes some of the experiences of those working in the field.

£13.99 0–86242–171–3

The 36-Hour Day: A family guide to caring at home for people with Alzheimer's disease and other confusional illnesses
Nancy L Mace and Peter V Rabins MD

This highly successful, sensitive guide carries information on the medical, legal, financial and emotional aspects of caring, combining practical advice with specific examples.

Co-published with Headway

£12.99 0–340–56382–6

Marevan: warfarin sodium 48
mebendazole 128
Medised: antihistamines 53
mefloquine 128
Melleril: thioridazine 70
menadiol sodium phosphate tablets:
    vitamin K 122
Menophase: oestrogen and
    progestogen (cyclic) 81
menthol: rubefacients 110
Menthol and Wintergreen
    Embrocation: rubefacients 110
Merbentyl: dicycloverine
    hydrochloride 33
mesalazine 34
metformin 81
methyl salicylate: rubefacients 110
methyldopa 46
metoprolol tartrate 46
Metrogel: metronidazole 114
metronidazole 114, 132
miconazole 132
Micronor: progestogen 82
Migrafen: ibuprofen-containing
    medicines 64
Milk of Magnesia: magnesium-
    containing antacids 31
    osmotic laxatives 33
Mintec: peppermint oil 35
misoprostol 34
Moduretic: hydrochlorothiazide 88
Mogadon: nitrazepam 69
Moisture-Eyes: hypromellose 105
Molcer: docusate sodium 105
monoamine oxidase inhibitors *see*
    MAOI drugs
Monotrim: trimethoprim 133
Monovent: terbutaline sulphate 56
mood-altering drugs 64
morphine-containing medicines 64
Motilium: domperidone 67
Movicol: osmotic laxatives 33
MST Continus: morphine-containing
    medicines 64
Mucogel: aluminium and magnesium
    antacids 31
Mu-cron: sympathomimetics 54

multivitamin preparations 120, 121,
    122

nadolol 46
naftidrofuryl oxalate 47
Naprosyn: naproxen 97
naproxen 97
Natramid: indapamide 45
Natrilix SR: indapamide 45
Navidrex: cyclopenthiazide 88
Nedised: analgesics 52
Neo-Cortef: neomycin sulphate 132
Neo-Mercazole: carbimazole 80
neomycin 128
neomycin sulphate 132
Neo-NaClex: bendroflumethiazide 87
neuroleptic drugs 65
Neutrogena Long Lasting Dandruff
    Control: ketoconazole 113
nicardipine hydrochloride 47
nicotinic acid derivatives 47
nifedipine 47
Nifensar: nifedipine 47
Niferex-150: iron salts 119
Night Nurse: analgesics 52
    antihistamines 53
Nindaxa: indapamide 45
nitrazepam 69
Nitrocontin: glyceryl trinitrate 45
Nitrolingual Pumpspray: glyceryl
    trinitrate 45
Nivaquine: antiprotozoals 128
Nizoral: ketoconazole 113
Nizoral Dandruff Shampoo:
    ketoconazole 113
non-steroidal anti-inflammatory drugs
    see NSAIDs
Normacol: bulk-forming laxatives 32
Normax: softeners (laxatives) 32
    stimulant laxatives 32
Novaprin: ibuprofen-containing
    medicines 94
NSAIDs (non-steroidal anti-
    inflammatory drugs) 94, 95, 97
Nuelin: theophylline 56
Nu-K: potassium salts 119
Nurofen: ibuprofen-containing